STO S

CORONARY!

ALSO BY DAVID T. NASH, M.D.

Dr. Nash's Natural Diet Book

CORONARY!

Prediction and Prevention

DAVID T. NASH, M.D.

CHARLES SCRIBNER'S SONS / NEW YORK

Library of Congress Cataloging in Publication Data
Nash, David T
    Coronary!
    Includes index.
    1. Coronary heart disease. 2. Coronary heart
disease—Prevention. I. Title.
RC685.C6N34   616.1'23'05   78-13099
ISBN 0-684-15820-5

1 3 5 7 9 11 13 15 17 19   H/C   20 18 16 14 12 10 8 6 4 2

Printed in the United States of America

Material on smoking, in Chapter 6, taken from "If You
Want To Give Up Cigarettes", "When a Woman Smokes",
"Danger", and "The Decision Is Yours", is reprinted
with the permission of the American Cancer Society.

"Metropolitan's Desirable Weight Tables" are reprinted
courtesy of the Metropolitan Life Insurance Company.

The tables in Appendix 2 are reprinted from CORONARY RISK
HANDBOOK, © American Heart Association, with the permission
of William B. Kannel, M.D., and the American Heart Association.

TO MY FAMILY,

*whose criticisms and concern have been
pivotal in my maturation*

ACKNOWLEDGMENTS

"If I have seen further it is by standing upon the shoulders of Giants."*

In the preparation of this book I have benefited from the efforts of a large number of my teachers, students, and most of all my patients. The editorial talents of Iris Blumenthal made it possible for even the most esoteric of scientific concepts in this manuscript to be understood by any literate person. Sheila Crowley and John Mitchell read and edited some of the earliest drafts; their travail improved the final product. Several health professionals, including Stella Siroka, Sue O'Hara, Dr. Phyllis Hollenback, Sue Vail, and Dr. Pat Randall read portions of the manuscript and gave me competent, constructive criticism. Dr. William B. Kannel was kind enough to review the final draft. Finally, Susanne Kirk, my editor at Scribners, gave encouragement and succor to a fledgling author.

*Sir Isaac Newton in a letter to Robert Hooke February 5, 1675.

CONTENTS

ix

CORONARY!

Introduction

Heart disease means any abnormality that interferes with the normal functioning of the heart. This book deals entirely with atherosclerotic heart disease caused by narrowing of the coronary arteries, the arteries that nourish the heart. I specifically exclude other forms of heart disease (congenital and rheumatic, for instance) because these forms are much less common, less relevant to adults, and very different from atherosclerotic heart disease in their prediction and treatment.

The time has come for an accurate but readable book that provides up-to-date information on heart disease—how to recognize and treat it and, more important, how to predict and prevent it. Unfortunately, most heart books now available fall short of this goal. They are either scientifically valid but dull and geared to the medically sophisticated reader, or lively and well written but full of inaccuracies and misleading generalizations. My aim here is to provide vital information that is current, medically correct, and understandable to the lay reader.

Many physicians are reluctant or too busy to answer their patients' questions. In this book I discuss at length some of the most important topics my patients raise with me. I give candid answers from my standpoint as a physician actively involved in patient care and research into the causes and treatment of heart disease. Readers will learn what a heart attack is actually like, thus familiarizing themselves with an event that at least 1 million Americans experience yearly. The ensuing complications will also be described. I will deal with the symptoms produced by heart disease as well as current diagnostic techniques such as coronary arteriography, undoubtedly the most accurate method available to investigate the anatomy of the coronary arteries.

The treatment of coronary heart disease, including the pros and cons of open-heart surgery, is discussed. A complete analysis of the methods used to decide who needs such surgery provides insight into this difficult judgment.

To reduce the risks of heart disease, much more than valid information is needed. We must in many cases modify our behavior and total life-style. As a help toward that goal, the book includes a complete program to stop smoking, utilizing a variety of successfully proven techniques. Diet and exercise information are presented as well in precise detail. By the time you complete this book you will know how to help insure your own successful program of preventive maintenance. You will have learned the way to better heart health.

CHAPTER ONE

Prevention of Heart Disease:
It's Up to You

This is a book about coronary atherosclerosis. The term *atherosclerosis* means hardening of the arteries, and coronary atherosclerosis is the form of the disease that affects the arteries that nourish the heart.

Most authorities believe that the process of atherosclerosis, once it reaches an advanced stage, is relentless and inexorable. The vital arteries that supply oxygen to the heart and brain gradually become narrower—a narrowing that interferes with the flow of blood and impairs the function of the affected organ.

Possibly you are already developing the kind of heart disease called coronary atherosclerosis. Tragically, the majority of people so afflicted do not know it. What is worse, neither do their doctors. The simple truth is that most adults in affluent societies have varying degrees of atherosclerosis and few early symptoms. If nothing bothers you, why worry—right? Wrong! The first symptom may be a heart attack or a stroke or sudden death. Despite a $100 billion medical establishment, the majority of deaths in the United States are related to atherosclerosis. Many who escape sudden death from this disease linger on, helplessly disabled by stroke, neglected and alone in the back hall of some nondescript nursing home.

How can coronary or other atherosclerosis progress unnoticed? Simply: the early phases of many so-called degenerative diseases are insidious, and symptoms often occur only very late in the course of the disease. Autopsies performed on American soldiers killed at an average age of twenty-two during the Korean and Vietnamese wars revealed that a high proportion exhibited narrowing of the coronary arteries, which feed the heart. These soldiers experienced no heart symptoms. But they did have coronary atherosclerosis, and had they lived longer, many eventually would have developed symptoms. Interestingly enough, autopsies performed on Korean and Vietnamese soldiers of comparable ages did not show significant coronary atherosclerosis.

Fatal heart attacks and strokes (caused by a narrowing of the arteries that nourish the brain) are not, as the ancients believed, the wrath of a vengeful god who suddenly strikes down a victim. Rather they are caused by the narrowing of inner walls of arteries resulting from a gradual accumulation of excessive fatty materials. Although there is a great deal we do not know about this subject, research continues to advance. One of the purposes of this book is to analyze recent research findings that are important for all of us and to discuss the scientific investigations, some which I personally have had the opportunity to take part in.

Complete accord has not been reached by all experts, of course. There is, nonetheless, enough available information to enable you to predict and reduce your risk of heart disease and stroke. You may then choose the actions that are appropriate to your situation and establish your own game plan. For those who are at a high risk level but still symptom-free, it makes sense to start a program of prevention and reversal. I believe we can retard and reverse the progress of atherosclerosis. This view is not universally accepted by physicians, but there is solid evidence in its favor.

Before considering how to prevent or reverse heart disease, however, an overview of the problem of coronary atherosclerosis may be useful. Despite well-trained physicians, coronary-care units, open-heart surgical teams, and the best-financed medical research facilities in the history of mankind, 1 million Americans suffer cardiac deaths each year, about half from acute heart attack, the remainder from heart failure, stroke, and the ravages of hypertension. Equally frightening is the knowledge that the deaths from coronary atherosclerosis are but the tip of the iceberg. The rest of the iceberg is the millions afflicted with atherosclerosis who do not die—who suffer strokes and loss of function to the legs, kidneys, and other organs because of hardening of the arteries. The damage thus done to the body is usually permanent and often disabling. In 1977 cardiovascular (heart and blood vessel) diseases alone cost the American people more than $27 billion. Physicians' fees accounted for $3 billion, hospitals cost $14 billion, and drugs $2 billion. American workers lost an additional $8 billion because of disability caused by cardiovascular diseases. And obviously we cannot measure many of the losses caused by the disabling symptoms of heart disease. How can we quantify the effect of a strict proscription of sexual intercourse? How do we assess the impact on a forty-year-old truck driver who, after recovering from a near-fatal heart attack, learns that he can never drive a truck again? He faces two unsatisfactory alternatives: a lower paying job, for which he will have to be retrained, or reliance on his wife or the welfare system for his family's income. We can count the number of days lost to industry because of heart disease, but the devastating effects on the victim are harder to estimate.

Strangely enough, the prevention of cardiovascular disease has received little but lip service from most physicians. This situation has several origins. Many doctors are unconvinced that any attempt to reduce risk factors is warranted. Others concern themselves entirely with the evaluation and alleviation of symptoms and consider preventive approaches the domain of the local health department. Newer evidence that atherosclerosis can be controlled is considered the product of ivory-tower medicine. Furthermore, physicians are people, and they often seek the path of least resistance; it is difficult for them to persuade patients to change their eating, smoking, and leisure-time habits.

In the final analysis, prevention of cardiovascular disease is possible only if you take the initiative yourself. You must be actively involved in maintaining your own health; you cannot afford the luxury of leaving the matter entirely up to your doctor, your local health department, or a federally administered sickness-oriented industry. Americans have the most expensive health establishment in the world, but prevention of disease has a low priority. Therefore, no real alternative to personal responsibility exists. The buck stops with you.

If you are going to take responsibility for preventing heart disease, you need to understand considerably more about the subject. How much do you really know about your own heart? In the simplest terms, the heart, the greatest muscle of the body, provides the force necessary to sustain circulation. The heart is a pump, but it is unlike any pump you have ever seen. No manufactured pump can exceed its specifications. Each day your heart beats a hundred thousand times and moves forty-three hundred gallons of blood through the body's circulatory system—almost four times the amount of gasoline your car uses in a whole year. Amazingly, your heart can double or triple its output when called upon to do so. It maintains the pressure through sixty thousand miles of blood vessels.

The heart pump is a muscular tube that is subdivided into four chambers. Blood coming from the tissues enters one of the chambers, called the right atrium. The blood that arrives is bluish in color because it has become deoxygenated, having delivered much of its oxygen. It has reached the heart via the veins, the thin-walled tubes that gradually merge into the larger channels that eventually return to the heart the exact amount of blood previously pumped into the body.

The right atrium in turn empties into the right ventricle, from which blood is pumped into the lungs. Here the blood is reoxygenated, and carbon dioxide (cellular waste removed from the tissues) is released for exhalation. The blood from the lungs returns to the heart, entering the left atrium. From there it is sent to the left ventricle, the thick-walled chamber that provides enough mechanical force to propel the blood through the arteries. It is the arterial system that transports blood to the tissues.

The main artery leaving the left ventricle is called the aorta. The first branches of the aorta are the coronary arteries, which nourish the heart itself. Thus, the heart receives its own nutrition before the rest of the body—which is important, because the heart will fail if deprived of oxygen. But first it must pump out its blood; it cannot use any of the oxygen in the blood within its cavity. If it could, there would always be more than enough oxygen, and the problem of coronary-artery atherosclerosis would become an exotic medical problem. Unfortunately, the heart does depend on the coronary arteries.

Of the two main coronary arteries, the right and the left, the left divides into two major branches: the left circumflex and the left anterior descending. The latter nourishes the front of the heart wall and is so important that cardiologists refer to specimens severely obstructed by atherosclerosis as "widow makers." When cardiologists discuss coronary-artery disease they usually refer to these three vessels—the right coronary artery, the left circumflex, and the left anterior descending.

In general, heart symptoms do not occur until more than half of the passageway (the lumen) of the coronary artery is blocked. Some patients have a significant obstruction of only one coronary artery, others have two, and the most unfortunate have obstruction of three vessels. The more arteries involved, the more bleak the long-range outlook. Some branches are more important than others; narrowing in a small artery is less important than in a large one.

Authorities estimate that almost five thousand heart attacks occur every day in the United States. Of those victims who die, about half never reach the hospital. But heart-attack statistics are misleading. Many heart attacks go completely unrecognized. The patient may later recall a few symptoms that seemed to be indigestion or flu. Some of these patients have actually seen a physician who completely missed the diagnosis. Such an error is possible, even likely, because no two people experience the symptoms identically, and some symptoms are very atypical. The patient may even have no symptoms. The heart attack can occur during sleep and never awaken him. Only many months or years later can the episode be diagnosed by the telltale evidence seen on an electrocardiogram (an electrical recording of the heartbeat). In almost all instances of so-called silent heart attack, the physician who first saw the patient failed to recommend appropriate tests or electrocardiograms. The following case history illustrates delayed diagnosis and its possible consequences.

John was a forty-year-old auto mechanic who had been entirely well until six weeks before he came to see me. He had first noted a sudden onset of severe pain in his jaw while lifting a transmission from a car he was repairing. He felt a little nauseated and breathless but attributed that to smoking two packs of cigarettes a day. He had to stop what he was doing and sit down for a few moments. Since it was late in the day, John knew he would not have time to finish the job, so he decided to leave work somewhat early.

At home, John's wife had prepared his favorite meal: a full-pound porterhouse steak, French fries, and apple pie à la mode. After dinner he drank two glasses of milk and ate several chocolate-chip cookies. As he enjoyed the last cigarette of the day, his chest felt quite full, and he was uncomfortable when he lay down, but he attributed this fullness to the meal. Finally he fell asleep.

The next day John's car would not start, but after much aggravation he finally got to work. He had to park his car almost two blocks away, and because he was late, he hurried to the shop. The pain in his jaw struck him with greater ferocity; he noted that it eased off a bit when he slowed his stride. At work he asked two fellow employees to help him with the transmission. The day passed without further incident. The next day John went to a dentist, who listened to his story and then X-rayed his teeth. He could find only one minor area of decay but advised extraction as a precaution. John gladly agreed, hoping to relieve the recurrent jaw pain.

Over the next two weeks John felt increased jaw pain when he climbed stairs two at a time or had sexual intercourse with his wife. He also felt tired—so tired, in fact, that he scarcely did anything but work and go to sleep early. The jaw pains worsened. He consulted the dentist again, who referred him to an ear, nose, and throat specialist.

The specialist took some X rays and prescribed a narcotic for pain relief. The medication made John sleepy and interfered with his work and driving, but it did suppress the jaw pain. Yet whenever John exerted himself physically, the pain returned. It began to occur during the heated arguments John frequently had with the shop supervisor. John again called the doctor and was told that the jaw problem was probably related to a defective joint or to some obscure type of arthritis. The doctor then referred John to an orthopedist, or bone specialist.

The orthopedist listened to John's story and prescribed a neck brace to wear at all times. John went to the orthopedist's office every day, where a therapist placed his jaw in a contraption that would pull on his head by means of a set of weights. John spent thirty minutes and twenty dollars a day for two weeks. However, the jaw pain unfailingly returned when he walked briskly to his car after leaving the doctor's office.

John realized that he had been sick for almost six weeks and that he was always tired and short of breath. When he attempted to discuss his symptoms with the therapist, he was told that the doctor was too busy to talk to him. The therapist implied that John's symptoms were either imaginary or insignificant. John knew he felt worse and told the shop nurse at work, who referred him to me. When I saw John he was in obvious congestive heart failure, a condition resulting from the heart's inability to pump blood properly. When this happens, blood backs up into the lungs and legs and causes congestion of body organs.

An electrocardiogram proved that John had suffered a heart attack, probably six weeks earlier. Had John been appropriately diagnosed and treated, he might have avoided heart failure and recovered faster. I explained that the jaw pain was actually caused by his heart; it was a cry for help from that oxygen-starved muscle. Pains from the heart often occur in remote areas such as the jaw, neck, back, wrist, or even the upper abdomen. John had worked during the active stage of the heart attack and may have suffered more injury as a result. He was a lucky survivor.

Although medical mistakes caused a delay in John's correct diagnosis, John's own habits laid the groundwork for his disease. His risk factors, had he but known it, were a portent of trouble. He was a middle-aged male and a smoker, and he consumed a diet high in cholesterol and fats. His blood fats were probably elevated, although he had never been tested. John's eating and smoking habits contributed to his ultimate heart attack.

CHAPTER TWO

Cardiac Risk Factors

In an attempt to understand more about heart disease, the National Institutes of Health funded a long-range research project at Framingham, Massachusetts, in 1948. Over five thousand healthy middle-aged volunteers agreed to participate in a free physical examination and a series of simple tests. They were instructed to return for a retest every two years. Gradually, the investigators found several significant patterns developing in the people being followed. Many denied any heart symptoms, but electrocardiograms showed that they had suffered a heart attack since the previous examination. Hospital and doctor records were obtained and gradually a complete picture of the evolution of heart attacks and strokes became clearer. The study permitted a comparison between the original records of those who became ill and those who remained well. It soon became obvious that certain characteristics would help predict who would have a heart attack and who would not. The investigators named these characteristics "risk factors." Subsequent studies have broadened our understanding of the role played by risk factors in the development of atherosclerosis.

Occupying a major role among the risk factors is the level of serum cholesterol in the blood. Cholesterol is a fatty chemical (actually an alcohol) that the body requires as a building block to make sex hormones and bile acids for digestion. Cholesterol is found in all animal tissues, and in animals alone. Plants contain none at all. Cholesterol is measured according to the amount in milligrams in each 100 cubic centimeters of blood. The cholesterol level is described this way: ideal (below 200 mg.%), average or normal (200–240 mg.%), and elevated (above 240 mg.%). Some physicians claim that the normal range might extend to 250 or 260 mg.%, but at these levels the risk of having a heart attack is four hundred times higher than for levels in the ideal range. As little as 300 mg.% (1/100 of an ounce in 3.5 ounces of blood) is high enough to require treatment with diet and drugs.

Some people are born with a tendency to very high cholesterols. Their blood may contain over 500 mg.% and be resistant to treatment. Many will experience their first heart attacks as teen-agers and have strokes in their twenties.

Certain large population groups in Mexico and southern Europe have much lower mean values than the so-called ideal range of 200 mg.% or below. Among these groups coronary atherosclerosis is rare.

I do not mean to imply that a cholesterol level of 201 mg.% is unsafe and that 199 mg.% is much better. Actually, the level will vary from 3 to 5 percent in normal people. Physicians who understand this are able to minimize the variation by repeated blood tests over a period of time. The average of several values is a much more accurate representation. Alas, any cholesterol-level test is only as good as the quality control in the laboratory where the test is performed. Although most laboratories do a creditable job in measuring cholesterol levels, a few small laboratories do not. If a physician undertakes to perform the test in his own office laboratory, he must carry out repetitive quality-assurance testing.

More about cholesterol later; suffice it to say that a high cholesterol level is an important risk factor and can be measured easily and inexpensively.

Another risk factor is the level of triglycerides in the blood. The term *triglycerides* is less familiar than *cholesterol,* but it is almost as important. Serum cholesterol and triglycerides are both lipids, or fatty material. The triglycerides are fatty chemicals found in everyone's blood and have been studied extensively in the past twenty years. Patients with high levels of triglycerides have an increased likelihood of developing heart attack, stroke, or poor circulation to the legs. The triglyceride level is often elevated after eating, so the only way to measure it accurately is after a fourteen-hour fast. If you cannot recall fasting for fourteen hours before a blood test, chances are that you have never had your triglyceride level checked. People forget many details but seldom forget fasting for fourteen hours.

The triglyceride level is also elevated by alcoholic beverages and birth-control pills. Diabetics and obese people usually have high triglyceride values. Triglyceride levels are elevated by a high-fat diet or by eating excessive amounts of simple sugars. The ideal triglyceride level is under 100 mg.% (per 100 milliliters of blood); average, 100–150 mg.%; elevated, above 150 mg.%. Elevation of the blood level of triglycerides can occur with normal cholesterol levels, or both can be elevated. Unfortunately, much less research has been done on triglycerides than on cholesterol.

Most physicians still do not obtain triglyceride levels during periodic physical examinations, which denies the patient the chance to do something before the onset of atherosclerotic symptoms. I have discovered, in fact, that half the patients undergoing open-heart surgery at a major medical center did not have their blood triglyceride measured. Here is one area where an informed consumer can improve his own health care. Any physician can arrange for this test if you request it.

Another definite risk factor for heart disease and for the progression of already existing coronary atherosclerosis is high blood pressure, or hypertension. This does not mean that hypertensives are tense; many are not. Hypertension means only that the level of blood pressure is high. Most physicians believe that a blood pressure of 140/90 is the upper limit of normal. The numbers refer to millimeters of mercury pressure.

Why the two numbers? The blood pressure changes in a cyclical fashion; it is higher when your heart contracts and forces more blood into the already filled arteries. This higher value caused by the heartbeat is the systolic value. When the heart relaxes, the blood pressure drifts down to a lower level, called the diastolic blood pressure. By convention, the diastolic value is always written below or after the systolic value. Hypertension as a risk is fully explained in chapter 7.

Cigarette smoking is a definite risk factor, not only in acute heart attack but also in cancer of the lung. Almost everyone who thinks about it understands that smoking is a health hazard; nevertheless, people continue in this habit. They rationalize by convincing themselves that they are not heavy smokers. However, I define heavy smoking as over one-half pack a day. As few as five cigarettes a day has been shown to increase risks. I will discuss the risks of smoking in greater detail in chapter 6 and will also present specific techniques to help you break this habit.

Everyone knows that emotions affect our minds and our bodies. Stress is a factor in daily life. John Hunter, an excellent British physician, wrote over three hundred years ago, "My life is in the hands of any scoundrel who angers me." (His words were prophetic: he died following—and perhaps as a result of—a heated discussion.) Despite the fact that the role of emotions in heart disease has been suspected for a long time, the exact relationship of stress, personality, emotions, and heart disease is still under vigorous debate.

Two West Coast physicians, Meyer Friedman and Ray Rosemann, speculated on the relationship of stress and personality types. They defined as a "type-A personality" a person who appears to be under increased risk of heart disease. A type-A personality is very time conscious, always doing two jobs at once. In a conversation he impatiently interrupts a slow-speaking friend by interjecting the next phrase. In a restaurant he becomes furious if he must wait for a table. On the highway he is compelled to pass another car even if he is not in a hurry. Type A seems to be in a self-induced race and often goes through his limited life span as quickly as possible, fearing that he will miss something if he sits back and relaxes a bit.

Type A is in sharp contrast to type B, who has fewer heart attacks, tends to talk slowly, and never appears to be in a hurry. Actually, type-B people can be as productive as type-A people, but they do not seem so time conscious. They also smoke less and have less cholesterol. The role of type-A behavior as a risk factor is suggestive, but here again some physicians are skeptical.

The usual television stereotype of the victim of a sudden heart attack is the highly paid, hard-driving type-A male executive who succumbs at the peak of his career. This can be misleading: a study of a large industrial firm has shown that top executives have a much lower risk of heart attack than their subordinates. Possibly they have been preselected for good health in their competitive climb to the top. Another possibility is that once they succeed, they relax. The observation is valid even if the explanation is obscure.

Perhaps as a reflection of stress, people living in Western industrial societies appear to have a higher risk of heart disease than those who inhabit less developed lands such as the Indian subcontinent. And city dwellers have more heart attacks than do rural people (although there have been recent reports of a reverse trend). The roles of religion, culture, and early-life training are uncertain, but they probably have a significant impact.

Obesity is another risk factor. Almost nobody likes to be fat. Even those who play the role of the jolly, rotund buffoon almost certainly dream of being thin. But obesity does more than damage your pride and limit your wardrobe. Actually, there is a great debate on obesity raging among those who study coronary-artery disease, with some experts claiming that obesity does not increase the risk. They argue that only the high blood pressure, blood sugar, and blood fats that are common in the obese cause the increased risk; others claim an increased risk from obesity alone. Such arguments resemble the medieval discussions of how many angels can dance on the head of a pin. The truth is that people who are fat are at an increased risk; it is small consolation to be told that this risk is secondary rather than primary.

If you are a very sedentary person, then you also have an increased risk of coronary atherosclerosis—which means an increased risk of heart attack. If you do suffer a heart attack, your chances of surviving are less than those of an afflicted person who is physically active. We know that long-distance runners have a low incidence of serious heart disease. Of course, self-selection may play a large role in determining who decides to run as a hobby; the sicker you are, the less likely you are to develop the interest and skill. However, graded exercises for almost anyone are helpful and can be used to rehabilitate survivors after recovery from heart attack.

Just being a male is a risk; women are relatively immune to heart attacks. It may not seem fair, but there it is, an unassailable statistic. There are many theories as to why this is so, but we simply do not know. To complicate matters, many middle-aged men tend to increase their risks by denying their problems. Even if they know they have high blood pressure or high cholesterol levels, they often resist therapy; the macho complex interferes. Any admission of personal vulnerability is viewed as reducing their masculinity. Such men consciously or unconsciously suppress symptoms and may die dramatically because they are unable to change. It seems a high price to pay for unwarranted pride.

On the other hand, women's lives are changing today, and those changes are increasing their risks. Women are smoking more, taking high-powered, stressful jobs, and getting less exercise because of home appliances. They are also taking birth-control pills that raise the level of triglycerides. Perhaps these changes in female life-style will eventually produce sexual equality in heart attacks; perhaps not. As of now, however, men—particularly middle-aged men—are at greater risk.

In this age of transvestites and sex-change operations, can a man escape coronary atherosclerosis by opting for life as a woman? The answer is no. Despite the obvious difficulty in studying this personal area, certain information has recently become available. Some male survivors of heart attacks were treated with female sex hormones to see if this would lengthen their lives, since it was assumed that female sex hormones helped protect women. The men began to shave less, some developed breasts, and many lost their interest and functional ability in sexual intercourse. When the data was carefully analyzed, it appeared that the treated group actually died earlier than the control group.

The reason behind this seeming contradiction is the balance of sex hormones in men. According to recent research, the relationship between the amount of male and female sex hormones in men affects chemical changes that precede heart attacks. Some defects in sex hormone levels accompany abnormalities in the amount of sugar and fats in the blood.

Age is a risk factor that everyone knows about. Young people seldom have heart attacks; old people often do. The older you are, the more likely you are to have coronary atherosclerosis. The risk tables in the appendix to this book indicate how risk increases with advancing age. Of course, there are always exceptions. Some young hyperlipidemic people—that is, people with high blood fats such as cholesterol and triglycerides—have severe atherosclerosis; some eighty- and ninety-year-olds appear to have very little. Although age is a significant factor in hardening of the arteries, it is not the only factor, and its role is certainly not uniform.

A history of sudden deaths or of illnesses such as heart attack, stroke, diabetes, and high blood pressure in your family is another risk factor. Inheritance, or genetics, plays a role in the likelihood of your developing heart disease. If both your parents had heart disease or if their brothers and sisters developed heart attacks below the age of fifty, then you are at greater risk. Although you cannot change your family history, knowledge of the role it plays should motivate you to change the factors that can be improved. The matter has not been fully resolved, but research continues. (Chapter 11 discusses the genetic factors in coronary atherosclerosis.)

An additional risk factor that recently has received a great deal of attention is the increased use of simple sugars such as table sugar or sucrose in the diet. Certainly today it is hard to avoid sugar unless you carefully read labels and check such daily food staples as breakfast cereals, ketchup, and even sauerkraut. Although there is certainly no consensus that sugar as such causes heart disease, excessive use of simple sugars may be considered a potential risk factor, and it certainly contributes to obesity and weight gain in some individuals.

Another risk factor in the development of coronary atherosclerosis is diabetes mellitus, a disease in which there is a defect in the body's regulation of blood sugar. Victims of diabetes may first notice their affliction when they pass unusually large amounts of urine both day and night. The ancient Greeks recognized this disease. Eventually some ancient physician took to tasting his patients' urine and discovered it was sweet. Diabetes is a common disease in the United States, involving 2 or 3 percent of all adults, and it appears to be an inherited defect —although it may be brought on in almost anyone who gains weight massively.

The diabetic has a much greater statistical chance of developing coronary atherosclerosis than the nondiabetic. Diabetics also seem to develop the disease at an earlier age, and it often involves several areas in addition to the heart: eyes, brain, legs, or kidneys. Women, who are otherwise more protected by their sex, frequently develop accelerated atherosclerosis if they are diabetic.

Many diabetics are discovered by means of a simple test of the urine. In other cases it is necessary to test the blood-sugar level by means of a glucose-tolerance test. The latter procedure is easy and quite informative. The patient is requested to eat a large amount of carbohydrate-containing foods (i.e., bread, starchy vegetables, desserts) for a three-day period. After an all-night fast the physician has the patient drink a standard amount of sugar (usually about 100 grams, or 3.5 ounces), and the blood-sugar level is determined periodically for either three or five hours. If the sequential blood sugars exceed a level known to be normal, the diagnosis is confirmed.

The body's control of blood sugar is accomplished by a hormone called insulin, which is produced in the pancreas, an organ located behind the stomach. In the normal person, a rising blood sugar triggers an increased production of insulin, which in turn causes the blood-sugar level to fall. Among diabetics this mechanism is faulty: some produce too little insulin, and others produce insulin that does not work effectively. Blood-sugar levels of diabetics can usually be maintained in the normal range by injections of animal-produced insulin. Not all diabetics require insulin, however; some need only a weight-reducing diet, and others benefit from pills that stimulate the pancreas to manufacture more insulin.

Although a strict diabetic diet will often control the disease, a tragic irony lies behind this fact. For many years doctors warned their diabetic patients not to eat any sugar or starchy foods. Since that left only fats and protein, diabetics were usually on a very high-fat diet because the so-called high-protein diets are all high in fats. The most cooperative diabetic patients did as their physicians suggested: they avoided all carbohydrate and ate fats. Many developed severe atherosclerosis. Initially, the feeling among the experts was that the diabetes was entirely responsible. More recently, the hazards of high-animal-fat diets have been recognized, and diabetics have been encouraged to follow sensible weight-reduction diets containing starches. With a low-fat, low-cholesterol diet, even a diabetic can maintain normal levels of cholesterol and triglyceride in his blood.

Diabetes can occur very early in life, in which case it is often called juvenile diabetes and usually requires the use of insulin. Juvenile diabetics are frequently thin and have a strong family history of diabetes. Another type of the disease, called maturity-onset diabetes, is seen in patients over forty, who usually do not require insulin. Many maturity-onset diabetics are obese. Weight-reduction and careful maintenance diets will often control the disease.

Although diabetes is a risk factor for the development of coronary atherosclerosis, it may work this effect in an indirect fashion. The increased risk may relate to the coincidental abnormal fat levels (both cholesterol and triglyceride) shared by diabetics. Also, since diabetes is often a hereditary disease, it is possible that the gene for its development is located near a gene for the development of blood-vessel disease. The relationship of diabetes and coronary atherosclerosis may be based on the proximity of the genetic traits rather than on the blood sugar itself. Although we do not know the mechanism of the increased incidence of heart disease with diabetes, there is no doubt about the observation itself.

Another, little-known risk factor in the incidence of heart disease is the altitude at which one lives. A careful scientific study was conducted in inhabited areas of New Mexico where the altitude varied between twenty-eight hundred and sixty-three hundred feet above sea level. For the years 1957–70 the higher the altitude above thirty-seven hundred feet, the lower the death rate from atherosclerotic heart disease. The difference was limited to men and could not be explained by population shifts or ethnic background. One possible explanation lies in the rarefied air found at high altitudes. Daily activities at high altitudes require proportionately increased physical exercise, which may be somehow protective for men.

A minor risk factor may be soft water. In a variety of communities where only hard water is available, the death rate from atherosclerotic heart disease is lower than in communities where soft water is naturally present. Certain trace minerals in hard drinking water may affect the risk of heart attack. It is almost as though the heart pays the price for a cleaner laundry and sparkling glasses. The amount of research done on this factor has been small, and there is as yet no consensus among cardiovascular experts as to the significance of hard water.

If there is disagreement about hard water, then there is chaos about food additives. Many lay "nutritionists" have announced dramatically that the food industry is poisoning Americans and they often cite an increased risk of heart disease as part of their evidence. I am unaware of any specific scientific proof that food additives affect coronary heart disease. One writer recently claimed that the cause of coronary atherosclerosis is chlorine in the drinking water. Here again the evidence is unclear.

A controversy has long persisted about the use of vitamin E in the prevention of atherosclerosis, as though a shortage of this vitamin constitutes a risk factor for coronary heart disease. There have been many anecdotal reports about the efficacy of vitamin E in preventing and curing symptomatic heart disease. However, when the evidence is carefully examined by objective researchers, it does not appear to be very persuasive. Recent studies show vitamin E to be no more effective than a placebo in treating angina.

Several diseases seem to be associated with a higher incidence of coronary atherosclerosis. One of these is gout, the presence of which is apparent when the victim awakens with a sore and swollen big toe. Gout is accompanied by a high blood level of a chemical called uric acid. High blood triglyceride levels often accompany high uric acid levels. Although the classic description of the gout sufferer is a fat, pipe-smoking English lord, his swollen foot propped up on an upholstered bench, gout has now been recognized in people from all walks of life; it does not have a predilection for the idle rich, but it does appear almost exclusively in men.

Certain types of kidney disease are associated with very high levels of cholesterol and represent another risk-factor relationship. Treatment of the basic underlying kidney disease will often clear the excessive cholesterol from the blood and will therefore resolve both problems simultaneously. When the failure of the kidney function is severe, however, waste products usually removed from the blood by the kidney and excreted in the urine begin to accumulate in the body. They can be mechanically removed by dialysis, an artificial method of periodically cleansing the blood and thereby prolonging the life of the individual who is without kidney function. Unfortunately, many of the patients so treated develop very high levels of triglycerides in their blood. With the elevation of this blood fat, atherosclerosis often accelerates.

Many fat people would like to believe that their obesity is the result of defective functioning of the thyroid gland; this is usually wishful thinking. When low thyroid function (myxedema) is present, however, it can cause a marked elevation of both the cholesterol and triglyceride levels and is therefore associated with a higher risk of heart disease. A deficiency of thyroid hormone can also lead to high blood pressure and thus to excessive atherosclerosis. The lack of thyroid hormone is also linked to a condition in which the heart muscle contracts poorly and the heart enlarges and fails to pump properly.

Certain characteristics that have been found to accompany a higher risk of heart disease can be recognized by carefully looking at a person's face. One of these is a white line around the iris called arcus senilis (more fully described elsewhere). Another is a diagonal ear crease, a sharp, deep indentation in the earlobe, which occurs especially in men below the age of fifty. This does not mean that the ear crease itself in any way causes heart disease, but the two may be associated.

Several other factors have been suggested as being partially responsible for the development of coronary atherosclerosis, including various vitamin deficiencies, poor tissue tone, geographical location, infections, toxins, and even constipation. In all these instances it is usually not possible to exclude a relationship between some environmental problem or personal stress and the subsequent development of heart disease. When compared with the standard well-documented risk factors already outlined, these peripheral factors clearly are less important.

No review of the known and suggested risk factors would be complete without a repetition of the following disclaimer: we do not know the exact cause of coronary atherosclerosis. Most of those who work in this area believe that a mosaic of causes is responsible. We cannot say with absolute mathematical certainty that changing the risk factors will prevent or cure existing coronary atherosclerosis. No proven method exists for the cure of coronary-artery atherosclerosis today. Therefore, the best we can do is to use our present knowledge to remove ourselves as much as possible from what we recognize statistically as high-risk categories, and to make a realistic assessment of our situation. Chapter 19 will explain how to use statistical tables for such an assessment.

Before leaving the subject of risks, it might be instructive to describe a young woman who at first glance would not seem to be the typical heart-attack type. But youth, gender, and physical activity did not protect her sufficiently. Careful analysis will reveal that risk factors were indeed present.

Connie was a thirty-year-old woman with two children, a husband, a good home, and high blood pressure. She had been aware of some recent excessive weight gain and could not wear some of her more chic clothes. Her birth-control pills had elevated her triglyceride level, but she was not aware of it. She resolved to play more tennis, hoping that she could slim down painlessly while enjoying and improving her game. One day she noted some nausea and fatigue during a vigorous doubles match, so she stopped playing early. She assumed she had eaten something that had disagreed with her.

Chasing around the house to fix supper, arrange the children's various extracurricular activities, and finish some extra typing she was doing for her husband, Connie crumpled an empty cigarette package in her hand and suddenly realized that she had started a new carton that morning. This was her second empty pack. She then became faintly aware of a minor but nagging ache in her chest and back. "Must be growing old" was the first thought that came to her. She did not connect this with the earlier episode of nausea and fatigue on the tennis court. Shortly thereafter, the ache in her back grew more insistent, and she was aware of a squeezing sensation in her chest, just under her breastbone. "My bra must be getting tighter," she rationalized. There was a distinct sensation of a dull weight in her chest now, and a barely perceptible increase in the effort she expended breathing. She was not in any great pain. She was not short of breath, yet she was not comfortable, either.

The intensity of Connie's discomfort gradually worsened until she felt a viselike grip in her chest. She could not hide her distress from her husband: he noted her frown and the bead of sweat on her forehead. Connie grudgingly confessed to him and to herself for the first time that she was having severe chest pain. He took her to the emergency room of the hospital and thereby saved her life.

In the examining area she could not believe this was happening to her. By the time she had put on the hospital gown, her chest pain was so severe that she cried out. A nurse came in and took her temperature, pulse, and blood pressure. An intern began to fire questions at her.

Connie became increasingly aware that she was light-headed and that the chest pain was much worse. They had hooked her up to an electrocardiographic monitor, and an image of her heart's electrical activity appeared on an oscilloscope (a small television screen on which a moving beam of electrons draws a pattern of the heart's activity). The intern was shouting orders at the nurse now; both seemed agitated and concerned. Connie felt as though she was going to faint. She could hardly see or hear. Sensing the panic in the nurse and intern, she thought she was going to die.

Connie lost consciousness as her heart lapsed into ventricular fibrillation (an ineffective quivering of the heart muscle), her circulation ceased, and her heart no longer pumped blood. Immediately upon seeing the rhythm change and observing Connie's loss of consciousness, the intern applied a pair of large paddles to her chest. They were coated with a thick, jellied salt solution. He cautioned the nurse to avoid touching Connie and then administered a countershock current.

There was a spasmodic contraction of Connie's entire body. The localized electrocution of sorts had erased her abnormal rhythm, and she began to have a regular heartbeat again.

She did not recover consciousness for a while. When she finally awoke, she began to understand more about what had occurred, and she wept. "This can't be happening to me," she said. "It's not fair. I'm too young, and I'm a woman. Heart attacks don't affect people like me." Unfortunately, they do, and Connie was wrong. Women who have high blood pressure, smoke, and are overweight, especially those with excessive triglycerides, seem to lose the immunity of their sex to heart attacks.

Connie learned during her hospitalization that most people can be completely rehabilitated and that chronic disability and invalidism need not be the alternative to dying. She has fully recovered since then. She no longer smokes, her blood pressure and triglyceride levels are lower, and she is thinner. Perhaps another heart attack will be prevented.

CHAPTER THREE

How Atherosclerosis Occurs

It is important to know what causes a disease in order to prevent it or treat it appropriately. The genesis of atherosclerosis, as already indicated, is the subject of numerous investigations and endless debate. Its exact causes are still unknown, but they seem to be linked to the many factors that are outlined in chapter 2. This guilt by association is stronger for some factors than for others, but taken as a group, they are powerful predictors of the future. A common denominator, an underlying connection that would tie these various factors together into one cogent and convincing thesis, is elusive.

The best way to start looking for the cause of atherosclerosis is by examining the information that we already have. We know that an artery may become increasingly clogged with atherosclerotic plaques, which are heaped-up collections of connective tissue, fats, and smooth muscle cells. The plaques project into the lumen, or passageway, of the artery and interfere with the flow of blood. Normally the smooth muscle cells are found in the middle layer of the arterial wall; in atherosclerosis they migrate into the inner layer. If we could understand why the smooth muscle cells migrate, we could begin to unravel the mystery of atherosclerosis. Several theories have been proposed that suggest mechanisms by which the earliest lesions of atherosclerosis occur. In order better to understand atherosclerosis, you should know the structure and function of arteries.

An artery has an elastic wall, and the blood flow in the artery is pulsatile, corresponding to the pumping action of the heart. The artery wall consists of an intima, or inner lining; the media, or muscular area; and the adventitia, or outer lining. A single layer of cells, the endothelium, lines the inner surface of the intima. These endothelial cells control the passage of water and chemicals from the bloodstream into the tissues. The remainder of the intima consists largely of noncellular connective-tissue fibers. The intima tends to thicken with age and is thicker in men than women. The number of cells in the intima increases with age in both sexes. Atherosclerosis begins in the intima and is first recognized as a lumpy deposit—the plaques—that thickens the inner wall of the artery.

Separating the intima from the media is a band of elastic tissue called the internal elastic membrane. The media itself consists of smooth muscle cells that are contractile but are not under conscious control, as are the larger skeletal muscles of the legs and arms. The proliferation of smooth muscle cells underlies the atherosclerotic process.

Implicated in the formation of a plaque is a component of the blood called the platelets, small cellular particles that contribute to the clotting mechanism. Platelets also provide a stimulus for growth of the smooth muscle cells. When smooth muscle cells are grown in the absence of platelets, the cells remain dormant; animals that lack platelets do not develop atherosclerosis, regardless of whether the lack of platelets occurs naturally or is produced experimentally.

The first theory explaining the origin of atherosclerosis was suggested by the German pathologist Rudolf Virchow over a hundred years ago. Virchow's theory still has considerable merit. He suggested that the passage of fatty material into the arterial wall is the initiating cause of atherosclerosis. This fatty material, especially cholesterol, acts as an irritant, and the artery wall responds with an outpouring of cells that eventually can be recognized as an atherosclerotic plaque. Virchow's theory was supported by the later discovery that high levels of cholesterol in the diet and in the blood dramatically increase the incidence of coronary atherosclerosis. The theory gained momentum when N. N. Anitischkow showed in 1912 that he could create atheroscleroticlike lesions in rabbits by feeding them a high-cholesterol diet. The rabbit diet included eggs, milk, and butter. Anitischkow's experiment has been repeated all over America by the unwary under the guise of eating well.

Virchow suggested that injury to the intima in some way initiated the process of atherosclerosis. Russell Ross and Laurence Harker, working recently at the University of Washington, used monkeys in a variety of imaginative experiments to provide convincing evidence of the validity of this theory. They demonstrated that injury to the endothelial, or intimal lining, cells played a role in the production of the atherosclerotic plaque. Ross and Harker first studied the effects of platelets on the evolution of atherosclerosis, noting that platelets adhered to the area of the intima where the endothelium was injured. Eventually this injured area became raised—that is, a plaque. In monkeys with normal cholesterol levels, the injury to the intima healed. But in monkeys that had persistently high cholesterol levels, the lesions progressed and healing did not occur. Instead, a larger injury with debris and cells containing lipids (i.e., blood fats, such as cholesterol) developed. Mechanically injured arteries in one group of monkeys resembled the arteries of another group that was persistently maintained in a state of high blood cholesterol. Thus, definite evidence was developed that the level of cholesterol (in monkeys) can directly injure the intima and can inhibit the healing of injuries that have previously occurred, either mechanically or because of increased lipids.

A normal monkey has a cholesterol level under 100 mg.% per 100 milliliters. Generally, monkeys are vegetarians and do not eat foods containing cholesterol. After the Ross and Harker monkeys were fed cholesterol in the form of egg yolks, their average cholesterol level was 223 mg.%. This, interestingly enough, is the level found in the average healthy American. Most physicians would reassure you that at this level no dietary modification is necessary. Yet this amount of cholesterol caused a loss in the integrity of the monkeys' intimal lining. Platelet aggregations at the denuded area and the gradual production of an atherosclerotic plaque followed. Apparently, atherosclerosis can occur at blood levels heretofore considered normal or average.

A different theory concerning the origin of atherosclerosis was developed by the Austrian pathologist Karl von Rokitansky in 1852. He suggested that atherosclerotic plaques are the aftereffects of blood-clot organization (thrombosis). The clot adheres to the intima and is gradually converted into a mass of tissue that evolves into the characteristic lesion of atherosclerosis. Evidence to support this theory has developed recently. It has been shown that some of the usual components of a clot, platelets and fibrin (a protein that is the final product in thrombosis), are often present in the atherosclerotic plaque. However, cholesterol crystals and cells rich in lipid, which occur in atherosclerotic plaques, can also be found in organizing clots.

Although it has not been proven that thrombosis is the cause of atherosclerosis, the evidence suggests that thrombosis may play a role in the development of the more complicated atherosclerotic plaque. This role does not exclude the effect of high cholesterol. Severe atherosclerosis capable of causing symptoms of coronary-artery disease occurs only in those population groups with serum-cholesterol levels in excess of 200 mg.%. Thus, though thrombosis may be important in initiating the plaque, the presence of elevated blood lipids may be important in accelerating the arterial narrowing to the point that it causes symptoms. Both of these theories have their vocal proponents and detractors.

The latest theory, the monoclonal theory, was developed after the discovery of the role of the smooth muscle cell. Earl Benditt and a co-worker were investigating the development of atherosclerotic lesions in chickens and found that the usual method of feeding chickens excessive cholesterol was misleading. Although the chickens developed arterial lesions, examination with the electron microscope revealed that the plaques did not resemble human atherosclerosis. The researchers did, however, find a naturally occurring disease in chickens that bore a striking resemblance to human coronary atherosclerosis. This was not what they had originally planned on studying; but they recognized its importance, and thus they were able to observe changes in naturally occurring plaques in untreated chickens. The earliest change was the accumulation of a small group of smooth muscle cells in the intima.

Excessive cholesterol accumulation was not present in this early stage. It was likely that the few cells present had migrated from the media into the intima. In their new environment, these cells had multiplied and formed the small mound of tissue of an early plaque.

What was even more exciting was that these cells were subtly different from normal smooth muscle cells. They were smaller and had fewer connections with other cells. They also manufactured larger amounts of collagen (a protein constituent of connective tissue) and developed small cavities (vacuoles) when the chicken was exposed to cholesterol. These cells clearly differed from the tissue from which they had migrated.

Benditt proposed that the cells in question were monoclonal—that is, derived from a single predecessor that had been changed by a mutation, or hereditary genetic change. Sometimes, in animal tissues, a single cell evidences an unusual growth and multiplication pattern and enlarges into a mass of cells. Some event such as a mutation causes this. The cells thus produced are similar to the cells of a benign tumor. Benditt was able to study the intima of affected arteries obtained at autopsy in humans and found that the atherosclerotic plaques contained monoclonal cells. The monoclonal mutation becomes visible if the plaques are enlarged by the depositing of lipids and debris. In this way, cholesterol contributes after the initiation of the plaque.

The monoclonal theory provides a new mechanism to explain the effect of the risk factors in starting the atherosclerotic plaque. For example, there are chemicals in cigarette smoke that are potentially mutagenic. The effect of smoking therefore may be its encouragement of the original mutation that underlies the basic atherosclerotic lesion. The mutagenic chemicals stimulate a smooth muscle cell to initiate a new plaque.

The mutagens in the blood are carried by lipoproteins (the combination of cholesterol and a protein that is soluble in blood). Excess of lipoprotein may expose the intima to more mutagens. When known mutagens were purposely administered to chickens, the chickens were found to have an increased number of plaques. A chemical by-product of cholesterol itself may be mutagenic; the relationship of an elevated cholesterol to coronary atherosclerosis may be caused in part by an increase in the rate of mutants in the smooth muscle cells of the media. High blood pressure may exert its effect by increasing pressure on the arterial walls, stimulating the cells to multiply faster.

After the plaque has been initiated, cholesterol will infiltrate the intima and be deposited into the smooth muscle cells. After a while some of the cells die, and their debris contains a variety of fatty materials, including cholesterol. The deposition of cholesterol in and out of the smooth muscle cells enlarges the plaque and encourages the narrowing of the arterial passageway. Control of this fatty deposit in the plaque offers the best hope for the reversal of coronary atherosclerosis.

From dietary and lipid-lowering experiments in monkeys, we know that the lipid fraction of the plaque can be mobilized. Whether the cholesterol causes the plaque by its mutagenic effect on smooth muscle cells or merely enlarges an existing plaque by passive infiltration, lowering the cholesterol makes therapeutic sense.

The monoclonal theory is important because it represents a recent departure from traditional beliefs about the origins of atherosclerosis. The idea that the cause of atherosclerosis may in fact rest in some form of benign tumor is interesting. Although none of the theories we have discussed concerning the cause of atherosclerosis is known to be absolutely correct or incorrect, each provides us with challenging areas of investigation into the mechanism of this disease, which may suggest better methods of treatment and prevention.

CHAPTER FOUR

The Symptoms and Signs
of Coronary Atherosclerosis

Physicians make a distinction between symptoms and signs. Symptoms are the feelings that the patient notices. Signs are those physical changes that can be recognized by physician or patient and that provide clues to the diagnosis of heart disease.

Once symptoms are present, the diagnosis of coronary heart disease can be made by the patient himself. In my lectures to medical students learning about cardiology, I often use a saying that I myself heard as a student: "Listen to the patient; he is trying to tell you what is wrong with him." A careful history of where, when, what, and how the patient feels discomfort is all that is necessary. A good doctor diagnoses most heart disease by taking a good history. Given a little background, you too will be able to recognize the symptoms. Although I would caution that you cannot become a one-lesson diagnostician, you should be able to recognize a typical heart attack. You should also be aware of enough basic facts to save your life or the lives of others, if necessary.

The description of chest pains associated with narrowing of the coronary arteries goes back to William Heberden, who in 1768 wrote about a distinctive "disorder of the breast." He noted a "sense of strangling" and used the Latin term *angina pectoris* ("strangling chest") for the first time. Heberden's description was so complete that very little can be added two centuries later. Angina (most physicians drop the term *pectoris*) is the pain caused when the heart is denied sufficient oxygen because narrowing of the coronary artery impedes blood flow. It is similar to, but less severe than, the pain that accompanies a heart attack. Angina pectoris is a symptom, not a disease: the condition it signals can cause disability or death.

Although the pain of angina pectoris often occurs near or under the breastbone, it can be felt elsewhere, as we have learned. Atypical locations include the left shoulder, the back between the shoulder blades, the left wrist, the upper abdomen, the right chest, the jaw, the neck, even a tooth. Often the pain does not stay in one location but starts in the chest and then radiates to the neck, jaw, and upper extremities; it may be felt throughout the left arm or in only one location, such as the wrist. The symptoms of angina occur in such obscure places because some nerve pathways to and from the jaw and neck remotely connect with the heart so that pain originating in the heart can be felt in these parts of the body.

The pain of angina pectoris is usually distinctive and affects any one victim in recognizably repetitive ways. Often it feels as if a vise or a heavy weight were crushing the chest. The pain can be burning, but it is not usually sharp, and it tends to be constant rather than throbbing; it cannot be ignored. It is characteristically brought on by emotional excitement, eating a heavy meal, or strong or even mild physical exertion such as sexual intercourse, moving the bowels, or walking. All these activities cause the heart to work harder, so more oxygenated blood is needed to supply the heart's muscle. Occasionally angina may occur while resting or sleeping. These forms usually indicate greater narrowing in the affected coronary arteries and probably mean that a larger number of coronary arteries are obstructed. Thus, the angina is provoked by exertion or excitement and relieved by rest. Anyone who thinks he has anything suggesting angina should see a *competent* doctor promptly. If the pain recurs frequently, it demands evaluation, and if a person has never before had angina, the first occurrence should receive immediate investigation.

The pains of angina pectoris usually disappear within a few minutes.

If they persist longer, the patient may have coronary insufficiency, a state of prolonged inadequacy of the blood supply to the heart. Coronary insufficiency is an intermediate stage between angina and a heart attack. It is not always easy to distinguish between them, although a well-trained cardiologist using a variety of new tests can do so. The prolonged pain of coronary insufficiency is not associated with the destruction of any heart muscle and may be brought about by some other illness such as anemia or pneumonia.

If such chest pain lasts several hours, then it is likely that a heart attack (myocardial infarction) has occurred. The pain of a heart attack is usually severe and requires narcotics for relief. A sense of impending doom or dissolution often accompanies the pain. Most of the time the victim turns pale and breaks out in a cold sweat. Shortness of breath often is present. A heart attack indicates the death of a portion of the heart muscle because of loss of its blood supply. The dead section of the heart will not be replaced. Scar tissue will form and strengthen the area of dead muscle, thus enabling the rest of the heart to continue its work as a pump.

Once a heart attack occurs, many problems can arise. The most important one, which determines whether or not you will live and how well you will live, is the total amount of destroyed heart muscle. If a small area has been lost, the chances for complete recovery are good. If there is a very large area of destruction, then the outlook is far from sanguine.

Some heart attacks are accompanied by dangerous, potentially fatal changes in heart rhythm. These may result in the heart beating too rapidly (tachycardia) or too slowly (heart block). In either case, the heart can no longer function as an efficient pump. Heart failure may follow either of these rhythm changes. More than half the victims of heart attack do not live long enough to be admitted to a hospital because of lethal rhythm disturbances resulting in sudden death. The complex equipment of a coronary-care unit is of no value to this silent majority.

There are many symptoms other than pain that are likely to occur in patients with coronary atherosclerosis. The most common, and often the most troublesome of these, is fatigue. Patients frequently recall an overwhelming sense of fatigue as their only symptom prior to the first attack of angina pectoris. Fatigue is frequently the first early symptom of an actual heart attack. A sense of fatigue can precede the attack by weeks or months. Characteristically, it is only minimally relieved by a good night's sleep. Not everyone who has fatigue suffers from heart disease, but severe, persistent fatigue requires careful investigation.

Shortness of breath, especially after trivial effort, is also an important symptom of heart disease. Shortness of breath may feel like fullness or heaviness in the chest and is in fact often confused with angina pectoris. However, most breathless people are out of shape and do not have heart disease. A good doctor differentiates important from trivial symptoms.

Swollen legs are common in people who have histories of heart disease. The excess fluid results from an accumulation in the salt and water content of their circulation. Salt-free diets and potent diuretic drugs correct the condition. There are numerous causes for excessive fluid other than heart disease, including varicose veins, obesity, and pregnancy. Many women notice swollen legs just before their menstrual periods.

When swollen legs are accompanied by persistent coughing, the possibility of heart disease is greater than when either symptom is present alone. Cough from heart disease results from a damming back of blood into the lungs as the left ventricle fails to work properly. The resulting congestion in the lungs causes coughing, wheezing, and shortness of breath. Cardiac-induced cough can be misinterpreted as asthma by both the patient and the unwary physician. This combination of cough, leg swelling, and breathlessness occurs with congestive heart failure, when the heart loses its efficiency and cannot pump all the blood it receives. The excess blood accumulates in the lungs and legs.

Some patients do not experience chest pain but do have palpitations that result in an increased awareness of the heartbeat. Palpitations can be regular or irregular and often take the form of an extra heartbeat —a phenomenon that almost everyone has experienced. When, in fact, several dozen normal medical students had an electrocardiogram recorded continuously for twenty-four hours, the majority showed extra heartbeats. Repetitive or frequent palpitations, however, require careful analysis and should not be ignored. Although most are completely harmless, palpitations can sometimes be a harbinger of sudden death. A physician can distinguish between benign and dangerous beats by appropriate tests.

Anxiety and ignorance combine to produce one of the most unfortunate aspects of heart disease. Many victims rationalize their chest pains by attributing them to indigestion and reinforce this deception by self-induced belching. Nausea and vomiting may occur at the beginning of a heart attack and often mask any chest pain.

Finally, it is important to reiterate that a heart attack can occur without recognizable symptoms. The victim either recovers, ignorant of his condition, or dies suddenly without voicing any complaint. Three characteristics of arteriosclerotic heart disease are recognized by knowledgeable physicians: the disease is treacherous, the course is unpredictable, and the prognosis is uncertain. Once symptoms occur, heart disease can be treated, but repair and rehabilitation are inferior to prevention and robust good health.

There is a deadly serious parlor game I would like to teach you called Predicting a Heart Attack Victim. The technique is simple. With three simple clues, easily visible to the naked eye, you make an educated guess as to who is likely to have accelerated atherosclerosis. The clues are physical signs that point to heart disease. Although there is no guarantee of perfect performance in this guessing game, the odds are very much in your favor. The clues are: (1) a diagonal crease in both earlobes, (2) a white line around the iris of the eye, and (3) yellow, raised areas around the eyes. It is hard to believe that all these clues are in plain sight, right on the face. No great skill is required in the obvious instances, but experience helps in the more subtle forms. Once you have the hang of it, you can do it in a crowded bus. I have been impressed that most patients have not recognized their own signs. And all too infrequently are those signs noticed by physicians in time to start a preventive program.

The first clue, the diagonal crease in the earlobes, does not prove the presence of heart disease, but it may serve as an early warning. The second sign, the white line around the iris of the eye, is commonly found in the elderly and is called arcus senilis. When present in someone under fifty years old this sign may indicate too much cholesterol or triglycerides in the blood. Arcus senilis does not always predict heart disease, but its presence should precipitate a search for high lipid levels. As a basic minimum, fasting blood tests for cholesterol and triglycerides are mandatory. The third clue is xanthelasmas, or raised yellowish skin blemishes around the eyes or on the eyelids. Xanthelasmas often suggest elevated blood lipids. As with arcus senilis, xanthelasmas demand investigation, especially when found in the young. A fasting blood sample and careful review of the family's history of heart disease is inexpensive yet informative. The search may prove fruitless, but if very high levels of cholesterol are found in a young person, early treatment may be lifesaving. The following incident underscores the significance of xanthelasmas: Arnold, a fifteen-year-old boy, had recently noticed raised yellow areas under both his eyes. Since they were painless and his mother had the same characteristic, he simply disregarded the matter. Like most teen-agers, Arnold divided his time between sports and school. He was on the high school basketball team, which meant lots of running. During a game one day, Arnold was dribbling the ball when he thought a weight hit his chest. The pain was so severe that he had to stop, and he lost the ball. He was short of breath and was glad when his coach called time out. The pain persisted for several hours. That evening Arnold was hospitalized with his first heart attack. He had not yet started shaving. Arnold recovered, and his youth prompted a careful review of his risk factors. He was found to have a very high cholesterol level, as did both his parents. Careful questioning revealed that many family members on both sides had experienced heart attacks and strokes or had died suddenly. 2033202

Physicians label this genetic form of high cholesterol as type-II hyperlipidemic disease. Unfortunately, it often escapes detection until the atherosclerosis associated with it has become far advanced. Since there is a familial tendency to type-II disease, it is possible to diagnose it long before symptoms occur, by examining all the relatives of those affected.

There are many other objective signs for which a trained physician carefully searches. As soon as he sees the patient, he quickly estimates the height and weight. A short, heavily muscled, stocky fellow runs more risk of heart disease than a thin, asthenic man. The patient's general demeanor can also inform the astute observer: a type-A individual has a higher risk than his type-B counterpart. Recognizing type A is easy for the average person; so is identifying ear creases, arcus senilis, and xanthelasmas. Do not panic if you recognize any or all of these risks in yourself. Instead, resolve to investigate all your risks—smoking, blood pressure, and so forth—and modify those you can.

Most people are familiar with the physician's use of the stethoscope in examining the heart. A great deal can be learned by such an examination, depending on the user's skill and experience.

Although physicians have used stethoscopes for more than a century, only recently has the significance of certain heart sounds been elucidated. A recent development has been the description of a new disease, caused by a defect on the mitral valve (the valve between the left atrium and the left ventricle). This so-called floppy-valve disease is caused by excessive loosening of the valve's support. A clicking sound is produced. For years physicians heard this sound and misjudged its significance, until the relationship between this click and a variety of symptoms was recognized. Patients with the click syndrome experience chest pains and palpitations that may mimic a heart attack. Unless the physician is alert to this possibility, the patient will be misdiagnosed and mistreated.

The sounds made by the heart have specific meaning. A normal heart has two sounds. In a diseased heart, a third sound often is present; it occurs after the second, and its presence may mean that the heart is damaged. A fourth heart sound may indicate that the patient has high blood pressure. When the heartbeat is rapid, the presence of a third or fourth sound may combine with the two normal sounds to mimic a triplet or a rhythmic cadence. This combination of sounds has been called a gallop because it resembles somewhat the sound of a galloping horse.

Heart murmurs are additional sounds heard in the heart. They may have a musical quality; they can be harsh or soft and vary in duration. The location of a murmur and its timing during the heart's cycle help determine its significance. Some murmurs mean that a serious valvular disease is present; others are completely benign sounds with no significance. Murmurs can occur temporarily with pregnancy, anemia, fever, or anxiety. A quiet room and a well-trained cardiologist are most important in the evaluation of any heart murmurs.

All these signs are important; they provide the physician with useful information at no risk to the patient. There has been an unfortunate tendency among too many physicians to deemphasize physical examination in favor of tests that invade the body with tubes, dyes, and balloons. Such tests are useful and yield valuable information—but always at a risk to the patient.

The emphasis on testing has had a counterproductive effect on medical education. I find graduate physicians who can rattle off a series of sophisticated test results with ease but cannot properly examine a sick patient. There is no need to choose between a careful physical examination and appropriate use of sophisticated tests. What is required is more training in order to achieve facility in both.

The majority of patients require a thorough history and a careful, thoughtfully performed physical examination to initiate therapy for most symptomatic heart disease. Usually a medical program will sufficiently reduce the symptoms of heart disease, and further decisions can be made over a period of time. Close follow-up examinations will determine what additional technically sophisticated procedures are necessary. Make sure that your own physician is oriented to long-range preventive medicine as well as treatment.

CHAPTER FIVE

Cholesterol and Triglycerides

For many years it has been observed that atherosclerosis affects various groups in a preferential fashion. In 1916, a Dutch colonial physician named Dr. DeLangen noted that native Javanese had a much lower level of cholesterol in their blood than did Dutch colonialists. DeLangen later described how rare angina pectoris was among the Javanese and suggested a low-cholesterol diet as a means of preventing atherosclerosis. His report had little impact on the medical community despite the validity of his early observations.

Coronary atherosclerosis is also rare in Japan but occurs with increased incidence among Japanese-Americans living in California. The native Japanese maintain a very low-cholesterol diet and have a low blood-cholesterol level; cholesterol levels are higher among Japanese living in California. The rise seems to be accompanied by a corresponding rise in coronary-artery disease. Japanese living in Hawaii are intermediate between Japanese in Japan and in California in terms of diet, cholesterol level, and incidence of coronary heart disease.

The situation was also originally true for Yemenite Jews, those who migrated from Yemen to Israel. They had very low serum cholesterol levels and little heart disease. Once the Yemenites adopted Israeli food and customs, they showed increases in dietary intake of fat, serum cholesterol, and coronary-artery disease.

There have been many studies in which various populations have been compared. Middle-aged men were observed in Yugoslavia, Greece, Crete, Finland, and the United States. Those populations that had low dietary intake of fats and cholesterol had low blood levels of cholesterol. They also had a low rate of coronary heart disease.

During World War II there were several unintended nutritional experiments that reduced the incidence of coronary heart disease in deprived populations. The Russian attack on Finland brought with it a severe shortage of some foods; fats were especially in short supply. After several years of food (especially fat) deprivation, there was a notable decrease in the amount of coronary heart disease and atherosclerosis seen in those who were autopsied. During the occupation of Norway there were food shortages and an accompanying marked reduction in the death rate from coronary heart disease. The end of the war saw a return to the usual dietary patterns and a measurable increase in coronary heart disease. The correlation of a reduction in heart disease and a reduced intake of dietary fats was also seen in the Netherlands and in Greece, both of which suffered under a brutal German occupation that removed much of the available food stuffs, especially meat and dairy products.

An American physician, Dr. Isadore Snapper, observed medical facilities in China before 1940. He wrote of the rarity of atherosclerosis and of the difference in diet between the Chinese and Westerners. The Chinese were largely restricted to a diet based on cereal grains, which are low in calories and saturated fats. Observations on the low incidence of coronary atherosclerosis are also reported from southern Africa and India. Throughout the world, where an indigenous group has maintained a low-fat, low-calorie, low-cholesterol diet, there has been an associated low incidence of coronary atherosclerosis.

The suggestion that cholesterol is an important factor in the origin of atherosclerosis was already forty years old by 1948. After all, N. Ignatowski, a Russian investigator, had demonstrated in 1908 that he could produce atheroscleroticlike arterial lesions in a rabbit. Feeding these vegetarians meat, milk, and eggs, Ignatowski produced atheroscleroticlike plaques by converting the rabbits from their usual diet to the affluent American's diet. Another Russian physician, N. N.

Anitischkow, carried out similar studies, as noted in chapter 3.

Many scientists insisted that rabbits are not people, that cholesterol-feeding experiments in animals are artificial and cannot be directly applied to the normal eating habits of man, and that animal liver can manufacture some of its own cholesterol. This information was seized upon by those who really did not want to modify their eating habits. The belief emerged that "cholesterol doesn't count." This belief is patently false; when a low-cholesterol, low-saturated-fat diet is followed, the cholesterol level will definitely fall.

The effect of various diets on the blood-cholesterol level was studied by a Dr. J. Groen in Amsterdam shortly after World War II. Noting that a typical Western diet was high in cholesterol and saturated fat, Groen compared to it the effect of eating a vegetarian diet that supplied an equal amount of calories. The vegetarian diet consisted primarily of grains, fruits, and vegetables: all the fats and oils were of vegetable origin. Those who followed a Western-type diet maintained higher blood-cholesterol levels than did those on the vegetarian diet.

Vegetable fats are unsaturated; that is, they have places for additional hydrogen atoms in their molecules. Unsaturated fats can be monounsaturated (room for only one more hydrogen atom) or polyunsaturated (room for more than one additional hydrogen atom). If the diet contains a larger amount of polyunsaturated fats and oils, the blood-cholesterol level falls. Monounsaturated fats are neutral; they neither raise nor lower the cholesterol level. Saturated fats—supplied by meats, dairy products, and artificially solidified oils, containing all the hydrogen possible—tend to raise the cholesterol level. However, most fish and polar-area mammals such as the seal, whale, and polar bear contain unsaturated fats. On the other hand, some vegetable fats are saturated; coconut fat is the most saturated of all vegetable fats. In general, at room temperature saturated fats are solid, and unsaturated fats are liquid.

An interesting aspect of the saturated–unsaturated fat story is the role unwittingly played by American homemakers and the food industry. In the early part of this century, most of the vegetable oil used was liquid and very cheap. Cottonseed oil, a by-product of the production of fabric and fiber, was used in frying and baking. Cooks found that it vaporized too easily and that a solid shortening was preferable for baking: but solid shortenings were more expensive than oils. The American food industry rose to the occasion. A method of artificially forcing more hydrogen into the unsaturated liquid oils was developed, which meant that a more profitable solid shortening could be made from cheap oils. People were soon convinced that man-made shortenings were what they had always wanted. What was hailed at the time as a scientific and commercial advance was in fact the production of an additional health hazard.

The Framingham study of 1948, already mentioned in chapter 2, tried to help resolve the controversy over cholesterol. Healthy people were followed along as they became older and sicker. There was no attempt made to change anyone's life-style, the only real intervention being a careful physical examination and tests at two-year intervals. The subjects were able to eat, smoke, drink, and carry on as they pleased. Except for the repeated testing, they were like everyone else who lived in Framingham, Massachusetts, a middle-class commuter town. The study also showed that although there is no absolutely safe level of cholesterol, the risks are minor if the cholesterol is very low.

It is a commentary on the status of medical knowledge in 1948 that the best-financed study of the development of heart disease did not include triglyceride measurements. In fact, there were few laboratories then that could accurately measure triglyceride levels. Since many physicians now in practice were graduated before 1950, it is easy to see how they can presently be uninformed on this aspect of the risks of developing heart disease.

Another criticism of the study was the arbitrary way heart disease was diagnosed. The diagnosis was limited to people who had electrocardiographic evidence or symptoms of heart attack or died. However, the majority of people with narrowing of the coronary arteries have no symptoms. The researchers had not planned on measuring the coronary arteries themselves.

Another study was done that aimed at documenting the amount of atherosclerosis in the aorta, the main artery of the body. For the study to be as representative as possible, thirty-one thousand aortas were obtained at autopsy in fifteen large cities around the world. The amount of atherosclerosis was measured carefully by a group of pathologists who did not know where their particular specimens came from and were able to avoid prejudicial judgments. After the study was completed, it was apparent that countries where the dietary intake of saturated fat and cholesterol was high had more severe aortic atherosclerosis than did countries with low-fat dietary intake and low blood cholesterol levels.

Another study measured mortality rates for coronary atherosclerosis in twenty-two countries. There were large mortality differences, and they were directly related to differences in dietary calories, cholesterol, and saturated fat. The United States and eastern Finland headed the list. Middle-aged American men had four times as many heart attacks as did men from Yugoslavia.

There is a common defect in all these studies: coronary atherosclerosis was measured by death or by the symptoms caused. I personally planned a study that would measure the progression of coronary atherosclerosis in living patients using a technique called coronary arteriography. It consists of the injection of a dye material into the coronary arteries and the photographing of the arteries on X-ray motion picture film. One can thus see the entire anatomy of the coronary arteries in the living, beating heart. The technique is safe and quite reproducible in competent hands.

I had the advantage of having access to the complete files of a major cardiovascular laboratory, including the records of patients who had had more than one coronary arteriogram. I decided to limit the cases studied to those in which the first arteriogram showed definite coronary atherosclerosis causing at least a 50 percent narrowing. Cases were further restricted to those in which determinations of both cholesterol and triglyceride levels had been made.

Only 119 cases met these minimal criteria. The first thing I learned was that about half the patients sick enough to need two arteriograms had not had even a single value of cholesterol and triglyceride levels established. Remember, these cases were studied in the seventies, not in 1948! It is easy to understand the average doctor's neglect of these risk factors when high-powered institutions are remiss.

Carefully defining what constituted objective progression, I learned that 106 of the total 119 cases showed definite progression or an increase in narrowing of the passageway through the artery. The average interval between these arteriograms was twenty months, so the progression occurred rather quickly. There were thirteen cases that showed no progression during an average interval of twenty-one months between the arteriograms for these patients. There were marked differences in certain risk factors between those who progressed and those who did not. For instance, patients in the progression group were much more likely to have high blood pressure, to be smokers, or to have a family history of heart disease. The most striking feature, however, was the relationship of the blood levels of cholesterol to the likelihood of progression. More than half (54 of 106) of those who progressed had a blood cholesterol level over 250 mg.%, and none of the nonprogression group of 13 had a cholesterol level that high. Only 16 of the 106 progression patients had cholesterol levels below 200 mg.%, while this low level of cholesterol was present in 9 of the 13 nonprogression patients. The likelihood of this last breakdown being caused by chance alone is much less than 1 out of 200. Among the patients who had an ideal level of both cholesterol (200 mg.%) and triglycerides (100 mg.%), only 1 of 106 progression cases (less than 1%), but 3 of the 13 nonprogression cases (23%), had such a finding. This is a highly significant difference, and it points out the rarity of progression in patients with ideal lipid levels. The facts speak for themselves: a higher cholesterol level is more likely to be associated with measurable progression of coronary atherosclerosis in less than two years.

My study has also shown that we can predict the likelihood of both progression and nonprogression, utilizing easily available risk-factor measurements. I believe that we have reached the point where we can say quite certainly that cholesterol level is related to the risk of developing coronary atherosclerosis and to the risk of the disease being progressive once it is present. We may not know everything about cholesterol, but it is an unquestionably important risk factor. Much of what we do know is new, although some knowledgeable physicians will remain cynical despite any new study. Perhaps a synopsis of what is known about cholesterol will be informative. At best, it may help you to protect yourself from atherosclerosis; at worst, you can entertain your physician with your newly acquired knowledge.

Cholesterol was first isolated from gallstones by the French chemist Michel Chevreul in 1823. He derived the name from the Greek words meaning "solid bile." As we have noted, all animal cells contain cholesterol, and all have the ability to manufacture cholesterol. No animal must rely on its diet to get the cholesterol it needs, since it can synthesize it to make sex hormones and bile salts from two simple carbon fragments that are uniformly available.

You will recall that pure cholesterol is insoluble in water and that chemically it is a complex alcohol. For transport in the bloodstream it is combined with a protein. This combination of cholesterol and protein, called a lipoprotein, is made in the liver and bowel. Proteins are able to combine with both cholesterol and triglyceride to form four types of lipoproteins. They vary in their size, their density, and the percentage of cholesterol, triglyceride, and protein they contain. The amount of protein in the lipoprotein determines its electrical charge. This charge permits separation of the individual lipoproteins for analytical research because of varying speeds of migration in an electrical field. This test technique is called electrophoresis and is easily done by any good laboratory or even in a doctor's office.

The largest lipoprotein particles, called chylomicrons, are formed in the gut during the absorption of fatty foods. Chylomicrons can be found after a heavy, fatty meal in almost anyone, but they normally disappear in a few hours. In fact, usually after a twelve-hour fast no chylomicrons are present. Chylomicrons contain triglyceride but very little protein, and they have very little electrical charge. This means that they hardly migrate in an electrical field. Chylomicrons can be identified even without an electrophoresis test, because they are so large and light that they will float to the top of a tube of clotted blood. There is a rare form of a genetic hyperlipoproteinemia (too much lipoprotein or too much fat in the blood) called type-I disease, which is manifested primarily by a great increase in the amount of chylomicrons. The blood looks exactly like cream-of-tomato soup. If you leave a tube of this blood in the refrigerator, the next day you will see what appears to be a cream layer on top. Type-I disease can cause painful attacks of inflammation of the pancreas. It is not a significant risk for most adults, because it is so rare (probably less than a hundred Americans are known to have it) and because most of the cases are identified in children. It does not appear to increase coronary atherosclerosis.

The next major subgroup of lipoprotein particles, called low-density lipoproteins, contains most of the cholesterol found in the blood. Low-density lipoprotein is definitely implicated in the development of atherosclerosis. Low-density lipoprotein is formed by the breakdown of *very* low-density lipoprotein, a lipoprotein that carries much of the triglyceride in normal fasting blood. Low-density lipoprotein has a specific role in turning off the cholesterol synthesis or production in certain cells. Recently, a specific receptor site (or custom-made docking site) has been identified for low-density lipoprotein in cells. The lack of these sites may be the result of a genetic defect. If low-density lipoprotein cannot dock on its receptor site on a cell, the cell never gets the message to stop producing cholesterol. People with this type of genetic defect accumulate very large amounts of cholesterol in their blood and often die early from coronary atherosclerosis. They have high blood levels of cholesterol and normal levels of triglyceride. Their disease has been named type-II beta hyperlipoproteinemia (type-II disease) or familial hypercholesterolemia (too much cholesterol, because of a family tendency). Fifteen-year-old Arnold, who was discussed in chapter 4, was a victim of this disease. This is an abnormal state of endogenous production of cholesterol due to an inborn error of metabolism.

There are two forms of familial hypercholesterolemia. A more common one involves a modest increase in low-density lipoprotein and has cholesterol levels above 275 mg.%. A single gene from one parent may be responsible. Patients with this form of the disease may have half the usual number of receptor sites for lipoprotein. This form is frequently seen in people who have heart attacks in their forties and fifties. In a rarer form of type-II hyperlipoproteinemia, patients inherit the characteristic gene from both parents and often have cholesterol levels above 500 mg.% and yellowish lumps in their tendons called xanthomas. Death in the twenties is frequent in this group. These patients may have no receptor sites for low-density lipoprotein.

Some patients have type-II disease without any abnormal genes; they have high cholesterol levels because of diet. This is by far the largest group and may constitute 5 percent of the population above the age of forty-five. These patients can be treated effectively with diet and drugs so that cholesterol levels return to below 200 mg.%. Vigorous treatment is required, however, and too often physicians and patients are reluctant to make the commitments necessary.

Frequently, the most severe double-gene type-II patients do not respond even after compulsive adherence to the diet-and-drug regime. The tragic part of this situation is that it is usually younger patients who have tenacious high cholesterol levels and who are most cooperative. They know what is in store for them because their parents and siblings may have double-gene type-II disease. The one hope for this well-motivated and fortuitously small group is the development of newer, more potent drugs to lower the cholesterol. In the foreseeable future we may be able to lower any elevated cholesterol level through various combinations of drug, diet, and surgical therapy.

There is also a type-III hyperlipoproteinemia, which shows an increase of a lipoprotein that is intermediate between the low-density lipoproteins and very low density lipoproteins. Blood from patients with this disorder contains equally high levels of cholesterol and triglycerides. Fortunately, this is a rare type of defect and is easy to treat. It tends to occur in families, and the definite diagnosis can only be established with some very sophisticated techniques not usually available. Patients with type-III disease have a high risk of atherosclerosis of the leg and heart arteries and may show yellow streaks on the palms of the hands. Unfortunately, the presence of type-III lipid abnormality is not recognized until the patient can barely walk or has a heart attack. Until atherosclerosis causes symptoms—often disabling and permanent

—the diagnosis of lipid problems rests upon fasting blood tests on healthy people. The situation will remain static until patients and physicians are better educated about the problem.

The most common lipid abnormality is type IV. People with this problem have high amounts of very low density lipoprotein, very high triglyceride levels, and normal or modestly elevated cholesterol levels. Type IV is frequently found in patients who develop heart disease and say that they never had a sick day before in their lives. In fact, they were ill in terms of the fat in their blood, but the illness never was recognized because their physicians did not perform triglyceride tests. The problem remained biochemical until symptoms made it clinically apparent. Type-IV hyperlipoproteinemia is a common cause of atherosclerosis.

Type-IV people tend to be fat, and many have a tendency to diabetes. Some young women on birth-control pills develop this type of hyperlipoproteinemia. It can be treated by diet, especially weight-loss diets. Many patients have type-IV hyperlipoproteinemia because of other diseases such as low thyroid states and pancreatic and liver disease. There is also a definite familial tendency. Certain high-fat fad diets result in starvation and can produce a similar blood picture.

Type-V hyperlipoproteinemia is rare and may be a combination of types I and IV. It may occur in alcoholics and responds nicely to weight reduction and abstinence from drinking. For all intents and purposes, only type-II and type-IV disease are common causes of atherosclerosis.

The high-density lipoproteins are the "good guys" in this scenario and may perform an important function—providing a transportation system to take cholesterol out of the atherosclerotic plaque and carry it to the liver. Usually, people with a high level of high-density lipoprotein have a low level of low-density lipoprotein and a low risk of developing coronary atherosclerosis. The reverse is also true; those with a high level of low-density lipoprotein (such as type-II people) have a low level of high-density lipoprotein and run a high risk of coronary atherosclerosis. Long-distance runners have high levels of high-density lipoprotein and little heart disease.

The smooth muscle cells of human arteries can take up both high-density lipoprotein and low-density lipoprotein, which may contribute to the tendency for humans to develop atherosclerosis. On the other hand, rats' arteries take up much more high- than low-density lipoprotein, and rats are very resistant to atherosclerosis. Perhaps the differences in atherosclerosis are more related to the ease of uptake of high-density lipoprotein than any postulated species differences.

There is a great deal that is still not known, and more research is necessary. It is clear, however, that there is a definite link between the levels of cholesterol and triglyceride and the risk of heart disease. We already know that people who go through life with very low levels of cholesterol develop very little coronary atherosclerosis; and we know that when a group moves from lower to higher levels of dietary cholesterol and fat and blood cholesterol, they experience a dramatic increase in the incidence of coronary atherosclerosis and heart attacks.

We do not have to know the final answer to the riddle of atherosclerosis to know what we must do now. Each of the theories of the origin of atherosclerosis (see chapter 3) is compatible with the premise that lowering the blood cholesterol and triglyceride levels is effective therapy. The dietary means are at hand, and the drugs necessary for the resistant cases are currently under development.

Coronary atherosclerosis is an enigma, a mosaic of risks and causes. We have identified enough to begin specific treatment to halt its progression. Physicians responsible for the care of the sick cardiac patient must insist on therapy to return the lipid values to ideal levels. If the physician does not, then the patient at risk must initiate the effort.

CHAPTER SIX

Smoking and Quitting

Each year cigarettes kill more than 200,000 people, make 11 million others sick, and result in the loss of 77 million workdays. Assuming an average daily wage of $40, the lost work costs over $3 billion annually. Although more than one-third of the adult American population smokes, the existence of 30 million ex-smokers is encouraging. Many people from all walks of life have quit; you can too!

The surgeon general's report that smoking is harmful and the active campaigns of the Lung Association and the American Cancer Society have undoubtedly changed public attitudes toward smoking. Unfortunately, there has not been a corresponding change in public behavior. Several attempts to reduce smoking by means of the mass media have been relatively unsuccessful. Part of the problem is that prolonged use of cigarettes leads to a psychological dependence, and withdrawal symptoms (tension, weight gain, etc.) accompany any attempt to quit. Strong social factors may also encourage the maintenance of the smoking habit. Young people often start in an effort to appease peer pressure. Since smoking is learned, however, it can be eliminated by applying known principles of behavior modification. What you have learned you can unlearn.

Almost every smoker already knows that smoking is not good for his or her health. Cigarettes change the function of vital organs. The nicotine may cause a smoker to have increased heart rate. Irritating particles carried by cigarette smoke are deposited in the lungs and interfere with the organ's normal cleansing action; this can result in "smoker's cough."

Smoking is a definite risk factor for the development of coronary heart disease. The more cigarettes smoked daily, the greater the risk. The likelihood of developing heart or lung disease also increases with the duration of smoking. Heavy smoking can be defined as the amount of cigarettes that will prove harmful to your health. It may be surprising to most smokers, but this amounts to less than half a pack of cigarettes a day. That is usually less than the smoker's definition of heavy smoking.

Another reason for reexamining your smoking habit is the expense of maintaining it. Heavy smokers spend several hundred dollars a year on cigarettes. If the cost does not bother you, then consider this: in a year a two-pack-a-day smoker burns up the 5 percent return on an investment of ten thousand dollars.

Many personal advantages not necessarily related to health follow when a person gives up smoking. That persistent yellow nicotine stain on your fingers will disappear. Your dentist will see you less often because your teeth will not be quite so discolored. Your mouth will feel fresher. The food you eat will begin to taste as though it has been prepared by a gourmet cook because your taste buds will no longer be polluted with a tar that resembles asphalt. The chances are that you will cough less, experience fewer sore throats, and bid good-bye to that annoying postnasal drip. You may even stop snoring. You will become acutely aware of delicious aromas. Flowers and perfume will be much more pleasant. Enjoying the delicate aroma of a fine brandy in a snifter is a joy that few smokers know; it is almost enough of a reward in itself for giving up smoking. You will have enough pleasures after a while to balance what you give up when you stop smoking.

Many smokers would like to believe that there is little or no scientific proof that cigarette smoking is really harmful. When challenged by their nonsmoking friends, they always seem to remember an old friend or relative who "smoked like a chimney" and lived to a ripe old age. They often conveniently forget those relatives, friends, and associates who developed heart disease, bronchitis, emphysema, lung cancer, and cancer of the bladder—all related to smoking. Everyone assumes, and secretly hopes, that disease and disability will only strike the other guy. Statistics mean little to the average person; but remember, if you develop the dreadful end product of smoking, then the statistic is 100 percent for you.

If there are any residual doubts about what a smoker can expect, some recently published studies may be illuminating. The incidence of sudden death due to heart disease is 3.5 times higher in smokers than in nonsmokers. This difference tends to disappear after you become a nonsmoker; and if you remain a nonsmoker, then the risk of sudden death may eventually become equal to or even less than the risk of those who never smoked at all. This paradox of a lower risk for ex-smokers has puzzled scientists. Several explanations have been advanced. Ex-smokers have fewer other risks than nonsmokers. More likely the ex-smoker has adopted other health-related modifications in his life. Possibly ex-smokers exercise more and eat less cholesterol. In any case, if everyone were able to give up smoking completely, then this country would experience about 25 percent fewer deaths from heart disease, and hundreds of thousands of lives would be saved.

Although every smoker is different, there are certain aspects of smoking behavior that can be identified. You may not be consciously aware of these pigeonholes, but they exist. In order to stop smoking, it may be helpful really to analyze what kind of smoker you are.

Some people smoke because it stimulates them and helps them start their day off on an active, more productive level. Smoking tends to delay their sense of fatigue during a long, demanding, or even boring task. They may not even be aware of a definite lift. People in this group really are using the chemicals derived from smoking as a stimulant drug; they can be severely habituated.

Others smoke because it provides a break in their routine lives. They delight in the ritual of removing the crush-proof pack and sliding the white flax paper tube out. Carefully, they tap the cigarette several times, ostensibly to remove loose tobacco shreds, but really to have something in their hands. They usually have a specific, stereotyped method of lighting up, perhaps with an expensive lighter. Their pleasure is as much in handling as in smoking.

Most smokers claim that smoking is relaxing and provides pleasure. This probably is true for them, but it is a learned response, much like that of Pavlov's dogs. You see, despite thousands of experiments on smoking, no chemical capable of causing relaxation or sedation has ever been isolated from cigarettes. Possibly there is a sedative in cigarettes that no one has found; or possibly people relax with a cigarette because they are convinced that it will help them relax. Actually, just taking a break in the day's activity and making a conscious effort at relaxation is the major contributor to the sense of relaxation.

Some people developed their smoking habit by relying on a cigarette to cool their anger or as a socially acceptable response to an anxiety-causing situation. They may have a history of depression and experience a sense of reduced tension by smoking. If this recurs (by coincidence, initially), they become convinced that the cigarette is a good crutch to use when they are blue, angry, uncomfortable, or upset. The absence of scientific confirmation has little impact if you feel that a cigarette will help you. If you want to believe it, it becomes true for you.

Some smokers admit that they do not enjoy smoking and never did. They may have started as youngsters in an act of parental defiance or an attempt to appear older. The original motivation is no longer present, but they cannot stop smoking. They have an unbearable sensation when by accident they run out of cigarettes. This craving is no longer a mere habit but a physiological addiction; it must be approached as such if there is to be a resolution of their smoking.

Finally, there are smokers who smoke almost automatically, simply by habit. They often light up a new cigarette, only to discover a perfectly good one still burning in the ashtray. They light a cigarette from the stub of the previous one and put it down, hardly aware of what they have done. They find a lit cigarette hanging from their lip and do not remember placing it there or even lighting it. For all intents and purposes, they have become human smoking machines, and their habit has effectively removed any pleasure in their smoking.

Now it is time for a great adventure. You will learn how to stop smoking. It will be a tremendous accomplishment, and it will be your own. This book will only supply the techniques. I use the word *techniques* in the plural because not everyone succeeds by the same method. Long-range scientific studies have developed, tested, and proved a variety of methods, so use the one that seems most compatible with your own needs and habits. Mark Twain said that it was easy to stop smoking; he had done it hundreds of times. But all you have to do is stop once, and permanently. Having made the decision to stop smoking, you are almost there.

Some preparation is necessary before any major campaign, and you will have to build up your motivation. Pick a day on which you will begin your planning and a day on which you will put the plan into operation—a D day of sorts. For the latter, try to make life easy on yourself by using a vacation, a weekend when you have leisure time, a period when your work load and family responsibilities will be less. But do it soon. Chronic procrastination will kill any good resolution.

First, make a list of the reasons why you wish to give up smoking —reasons that are personally yours, not necessarily the ones you read earlier in this chapter. If you have no personal reasons, you are simply not going to persist when the going gets a little rough. It is a rare individual who will stop because he wants to reduce the ecological impact of his smoking on the atmosphere. Your reasons can be modest; there is nothing wrong with wanting to save the $1.30 a day that two packs consume. There will be more than one reason for most people, but if you have one good personal reason to stop smoking, you are just as likely to succeed as the person with a long laundry list of reasons.

The next move is to find someone to whom you can talk about quitting. Ideally, it should be another smoker who is a close friend, but it can be any friend or even a medical or religious adviser—someone you can touch base with if and when you feel the need to. There are several organizations such as the Heart Association and the Lung Association that may be able to suggest trained volunteers to help you. A word of caution is appropriate: not everyone is comfortable with the idea of opening up about such a personal effort to others. If you believe that you would be more comfortable without a partner, then proceed on your own.

When D day approaches, plan with enthusiasm. If you view the venture positively, you will be much more comfortable than if you approach it as a one-way trip to the guillotine. Now make a second list, including all the good things you will gain after you stop smoking. Mention what we have touched on—a cleaner, fresher mouth; greater sex appeal; reduced health risks. Add some of your own secret goals. And plan on rewarding yourself with the money you save. At this point, review your earlier list of reasons for giving up smoking. Armed with your lists, your motivation, and the dawn of D day, you are ready to start.

The following method, suggested by Dr. Donald Fredrickson, has been used extensively all over the country and has been recommended by the American Cancer Society. It can be carried out by anyone who is determined to stop smoking.

The first day is so simple that you may believe it is unnecessary. Do not fool yourself; deviations at this point mean more difficulty later. Take an 8½-by-11-inch sheet of good white bond paper, a small pencil, and two rubber bands. This is the entire supply of items you need to stop smoking. Write the date on the top of the sheet and make five columns. The first should be designated "Number." On it you will list by number each cigarette you smoke during a given day. The next column should be headed "Time"; you must record the time of lighting up each cigarette. The third column is labeled "Activity"; briefly describe here what you were doing each time you lit up. The next column is labeled "Emotion"; a single word or two about how you felt—happy, angry, worried, bored—will suffice. The last and most important column is "Rating"; here each cigarette must be rated as to whether it is one of the most important of the day, of average importance, or among the least important. Now fold the paper, wrap it around the cigarette pack, and place the two rubber bands perpendicularly to each other around the paper and the pack of cigarettes. You are all set.

Every time you want a cigarette you must take the two rubber bands off; spread out the paper; take the pencil; and fill in the number of the cigarette, the time, the activity, the accompanying emotion, and the rating that you would place on that cigarette. You must complete the same ritual every time you smoke. So that you are not tempted to be lazy or "accidentally" lose the pencil or the paper or the rubber bands, you must make one simple promise: unless the form is accurately and completely filled out, you will not light that next cigarette. If you really do lose the rubber bands, you cannot smoke until you get two new rubber bands. If you lose the pencil, it must be replaced. If you lose the paper, start a new one with the best information you can recall.

Every night before you go to bed, review the list by glancing at the number so you will know how many cigarettes you smoked. Before the next morning, decide on which cigarette you wish to give up. Surrender at least one—more if you are in a hurry and feel up to it. Some pick the most important cigarettes of the day; others give up the easier ones first. It is strictly a matter of your own preference. Each night, see if you gave up the resolved number of cigarettes. If you find that you have retrogressed, do not feel guilty. Lower your sights back to a safe number (always less than what you started with) and then proceed as if no slips had occurred. The record of your smoking is to help you stop smoking and has no other purpose.

As you continue the gradual-reduction method, you will reach a point at which you are within a few cigarettes of total cessation. Once you are there, it is often possible to go cold turkey the rest of the way. If you are having some difficulties in lowering your intake, there are a few tricks that have been helpful to others: stop carrying matches; always borrow a match or light when you want a smoke, but only after you have removed the rubber bands, flattened out the paper, and filled in the columns. Another technique is to purchase a different brand of cigarettes every time you buy a pack. Purposely avoid the brands of cigarettes you like; either buy one you do not like or buy brands at random. I had a patient successfully stop smoking after I convinced him to buy his cigarettes entirely by alphabetical order. It is a sad commentary that there are enough different brands so that you can go through thirty and never repeat. Always buy individual packs, never a carton. Keep switching the location of your cigarette pack to different places in your clothes. If you keep them at home or at work, continually find a new place for them.

During the time that you are reducing your smoking, you may experience unpleasant sensations, cravings, and anxiety-related discomfort. You should plan on a variety of ways to deal with this. Some very successful methods have been developed: if the early evening hours are especially difficult, go on a nightly walk with your dog or spouse if either is available. If the weather or neighborhood is not conducive to walking, try an indoor mall or a shopping center. If you smoke automatically while watching television, turn off the set and read a book. If you find yourself reaching for a cigarette, modify the motion and brush an imaginary dust spot off your clothes. If the late-evening tension is very bad, plan some activity that keeps you busy—indoor tennis, swimming, sex. For those of you who find a cigarette after sexual activity is your routine, have your partner plan on a fond, close, and lengthy embrace afterward.

Try some reinforcement ideas when your initial enthusiasm wanes. One common pattern is to eat more, especially the foods you like. It is not uncommon for a long-term, heavily habituated smoker to go on an eating binge during the transition period immediately after he stops smoking. Do not concern yourself unduly with this weight gain; concentrate entirely on the cessation of smoking. However, it does help to have a large variety of low-calorie snack foods easily available. You can store cleaned and cut-up pieces of carrots and celery in the refrigerator. Some people develop a sweet tooth, so frequent servings of fruit as a dessert or snack are helpful. Rely on gum or hard candy to relieve your oral drives.

As the days pass you will find that you may still crave a cigarette, but the craving does tend to lessen. One day you may realize with a burst of euphoria that you no longer are smoking and that it does not bother you. Do not be tempted to light a cigarette to prove that you are cured and that one little cigarette cannot hurt. Some may be able to have a rare cigarette with impunity, but most of you will go right back downhill to where you were originally. The best advice is to leave smoking alone; get your kicks elsewhere. You can get a kick by considering that you have successfully stopped smoking and that 50 million Americans cannot make that statement.

Some smokers feel that the gradual method is actually harder than the so-called cold-turkey method. If you prefer an abrupt halt to smoking, there are a few rules that will help you survive the transition. First, tell yourself again and again that you simply choose not to smoke. Then, like those using the gradual method, pick a day to stop—even today, if you wish—and make a list of the reasons that you have for becoming an ex-smoker. Make another list of the things you hope to gain by not smoking. Plan on a reward for partial success and another for total abstinence after, say, two weeks. Be realistic and choose an affordable reward after the first forty-eight or seventy-two hours. You will appreciate and need it by then.

Some general hygienic principles have been suggested in the past, ostensibly to wash the nicotine and tars out of your system. Although scientific proof of their efficiency is lacking, these measures seem to help, at least psychologically: Drink at least eight glasses of water every day. Take a warm bath every night and a cool or tepid (depending on your taste) shower every morning. Give yourself a brisk rubdown with a washcloth and splash ice-cold water on your face. Drying yourself off with a turkish towel will invigorate your skin and give you a workout as well. Plan on increasing your exercise to the maximum with which you are comfortable. Walking is an excellent release; it burns some calories, and it is universally available. If you have not been given clearance by your own physician, do not attempt vigorous physical exercise. The fact that you are going to stop smoking does not in itself make you an athlete. Once you have completely stopped smoking, you can and should continue the exercise program you have begun and incorporate it into your life-style.

The gradual method of discontinuing smoking fails for some smokers despite their best efforts. They may be able to benefit from newer studies on the effectiveness of aversive conditioning, which aims at making cigarettes so unpleasant that smokers actively avoid them. One such method purposely encourages excessive smoking, usually one cigarette after another until the smoker feels ill. Some techniques include a fan apparatus that blows hot smoky air in the smoker's face. Some use a painful, but harmless, electric shock delivered while the subject is either smoking or told to imagine smoking. Another aversive technique is to have a smoker inhale every six seconds until he can no longer tolerate it. Still another form of therapy was tried by one investigator who required smokers to chain-smoke almost continuously for twenty hours before quitting. It may not be so difficult to stop after that kind of marathon.

An aversive technique can be potentially harmful in the presence of heart or lung disease and should only be carried out under the supervision of a trained professional who is experienced in the method. The advantage of this kind of conditioning lies in the speed with which it can yield results. Aversive techniques are an interesting new method of helping the smoker quit, but they must all be administered under carefully controlled conditions. It is not a method for the do-it-yourselfer.

An approach that recently has become commercialized is the education and group-support method. Groups are formed under the impetus of a local organization, and the members attend a series of nightly lectures. They receive encouragement and feedback from fellow quitters and also enjoy socializing. Groups are sponsored by the Seventh-Day Adventist Church, the American Cancer Society, and local lung associations. Commercial firms have been formed to provide such a service. Some make rather extravagant claims, and most have high fees. Their long-range value in helping people stop smoking has not as yet been firmly established. But it does make sense that if we can afford a $12-billion industry to encourage you to smoke, we should have an industry that profits by getting you to stop.

The techniques of transcendental meditation (TM) have also been used to help people stop smoking. The procedure consists of sitting quietly in a chair with the eyes closed and repeating a simple phrase or nonsense syllable over and over again. The meditator spends twenty or thirty minutes in this fashion every day. It helps reduce tensions and blood pressure and may well be a useful adjunct to those who are quitting smoking. Some other similar procedures have involved teaching deep muscle relaxation and having the subject imagine nonsmoking situations.

Most people experience some kind of withdrawal symptoms when they stop smoking. If they are given a plausible and reassuring explanation, they may tolerate the symptoms better. This was demonstrated in an interesting experiment recently. A number of student nurses who were all smokers were asked to take part in an experiment on what they were told was a new heart drug. In reality they were studied entirely for their smoking withdrawal symptoms. The students then were told they would have to give up smoking before and during the experiment. Half of the group was then given a placebo (a harmless, inert sugar pill) and was told that the side effects of this mythical heart medicine included irritability, nervousness, and increased appetite. The other half received no medication at all but stopped smoking in order to get ready for the heart drug. The study showed that the nurses who received the placebo and the explanation of the symptoms were able to stop smoking with a great deal less discomfort.

Some techniques have attempted to reduce the stimulus to smoking by changing the individual's environment and his behavior. One attempt involved the use of a special chair for smoking. All smoking at home had to be done in that chair. Gradually the chair was moved to more and more unpleasant locations, and smoking ceased.

A team at Harvard gave a group of smokers special timers and told them they could smoke only when the timer went off. At first, the timer used the interval the smoker was accustomed to smoking at, but gradually the interval was lengthened. Most heavy smokers were able to reduce to ten cigarettes a day with this method.

There is another technique, contingency contracting, in which smokers sign contracts calling for various rewards and punishments as they succeed or fail. A smoker agrees to set progressively lower limits on the number of cigarettes smoked each day. Any day that the number permitted is exceeded, the smoker must tear up a dollar bill for each extra cigarette. Within a reasonable period of time the smoker either runs out of money or stops smoking. This method is not dangerous, as the aversive methods may be, and it lends itself to the individual who wants to quit but needs an extra shove.

There have been several attempts to utilize various drugs in an attempt to ease discomfort and increase the success rate of would-be quitters. A drug called Lobiline has been used extensively for this purpose. It is an extract of an herb called lobelia, and it was used in the last century for people with asthma. It has the same actions in the body as nicotine, but it is less potent. Like nicotine, it can stimulate the brain and heart. Since it is much milder than nicotine, some physicians have used gradually smaller doses in heavy smokers who want to quit rapidly. There are no good scientific reports that it has proven valuable. Large doses of Lobiline can be harmful, causing vomiting, fainting, abdominal pain, and loss of appetite. It probably has little use for the average smoker.

Hypnosis is a method with definite value in a small, highly selected group of chronic smokers. The results have been good at times, but the technique requires a one-to-one situation with a highly skilled and experienced therapist, and it is relatively expensive. The hypnotist may use a positive approach, such as maintaining body health, or an aversive method. Hypnosis at present seems to be at best a last-ditch method for use in a small number of smokers.

A relatively new development has been the introduction of an anti-smoking lozenge. The lozenge contains asafetida, which has an acid taste and a garlicky odor. The smoker places a lozenge beneath his tongue before he lights up. The response of the taste buds and the rejection by people around the smoker act as powerful inducements to stop.

Finally, for the mechanically oriented, a holder has been developed with a variety of internal filters. As progressively more absorbent filters are used, the point is reached when little smoke and tar can traverse the filter; it becomes easier to go cold turkey and quit entirely. The technique is attractive to confirmed heavy smokers because they can continue to smoke. Like many of the previously mentioned methods, it can be successful if used with a compulsive progression by someone who really wants to quit. It has the advantage of providing a little extra help to smokers who have failed in previous attempts, especially if they view the special holder as a source of support. The device is fairly expensive but worth the price as a "security blanket."

A combination of the preceding methods is often more successful than any single technique. Remember that smoking is a learned behavior; no one is a born smoker. Will power is not required to stop smoking, but motivation is. Most smokers have had years to develop their habit and must not expect to stop effortlessly.

It is important to avoid any moralistic approach. You are not on trial; guilt plays no role in helping you stop. If you try and you fail, you are neither a bad person nor a weakling. If quitting were easy, it would not require writing about. The discontinuation of smoking may be the most intensely personal stress you have had to face. The rewards, appropriately, will be yours alone once you have become an ex-smoker. Good luck!

CHAPTER SEVEN

High Blood Pressure

As we have learned, high blood pressure, or hypertension, is a major risk factor in the development of coronary heart disease. It increases the risk of heart attack because it accelerates atherosclerosis and places an extra work load on the heart. Control of hypertension is fundamental to the treatment of coronary heart disease.

In 1964, at the Veterans Administration hospitals, Dr. Edward Freis began a cooperative study that proved that the treatment of high blood pressure would lower the risk of stroke and heart failure. His fundamental work underlies much of the newer aggressive approach to the treatment of high blood pressure that has evolved.

As you will recall, systolic blood pressure is the highest pressure level reached in the artery, occurring immediately after the heart contracts, and the diastolic is the lowest pressure recorded when the heart is at rest. A physician will usually diagnose hypertension if the blood pressure is persistently above 140/90. *Persistently* is a key word here. Everyone's blood pressure varies with activity and emotion. Several readings taken a week apart are much more informative than a single determination.

Blood pressure is measured with a simple, but ingenious, device invented by a Russian medical student in the days of Czar Nicholas I. It consists of a pneumatic cuff, or sphygmomanometer, an inflatable flat rubber bladder (the cuff that the doctor wraps around your upper arm, just above one elbow), and an attached column of mercury that reflects the pressure in the rubber bladder. The air pressure is raised in the cuff by pumping air into it with a small rubber bulb that is equipped with a valve. When the cuff is fully inflated so that all the arteries in the arm are collapsed, the air is slowly permitted to escape while the doctor listens with a stethoscope over the artery at the elbow. As the pressure falls, blood surges through the artery creating a knocking noise. The first noise indicates the systolic value. As the cuff is further deflated the knocking noise disappears, at which point the diastolic pressure is identified. Anyone can learn to take blood pressure. Once you have the hang of it, it takes only a moment to identify the different sounds.

What controls the level of the blood pressure? Two factors are most important: the amount of blood pumped out by the heart in a given time period, and the amount of resistance to flow as the arteries become progressively smaller and end in arterioles. The arterioles are very small, but they have a muscular wall and they control the resistance to blood flow. Reduce the output of the heart or reduce the resistance, and blood pressure will drop. The drug and nondrug treatments of high blood pressure work by affecting either of these factors.

What causes this fine system of control to get out of whack and result in high blood pressure? The most direct and accurate answer is that we do not know. Unfortunately, of the 25 million Americans with high pressure, only about half know that they have it. Of the half who know, only half are under treatment, and of those under treatment, only about half receive treatment effective enough to normalize their blood pressure. Thus, only one in eight with high blood pressure is receiving effective treatment, and 22 million are not.

Whom does high blood pressure affect? Everyone—the young and the old, the rich and the poor, the executive and the unskilled laborer. There are some categories—but they are not occupational—that are more likely than others to show high blood pressure among their members. But even if you fall into one of these categories, you will not necessarily develop hypertension. If you fall into several categories, it means that your risks are increased. Men below the age of forty-five are somewhat more likely to develop hypertension than women, but women catch up as they grow older. Blacks are more likely than whites to have high blood pressure. Heavy people are more often hypertensive than thin people. If either or both of your parents have high blood pressure, you are more likely to develop it. Heavy use of salt tends to favor hypertension's development, as does the use of birth-control pills.

The problem is compounded by the complete lack of symptoms in the majority of hypertensives, especially early in the disease. Most people with high blood pressure feel well, and by the time symptoms appear, the disease may be causing complications. Symptoms, when present, include headache, nose bleeds, excessive fatigue, and breathlessness. It is not practical to rely on symptoms to diagnose high blood pressure, since they may be caused by diseases other than hypertension. The only definite diagnosis is measurement of the blood pressure itself. Waiting for symptoms is courting disaster, because high blood pressure can kill or maim you.

Many years ago the very mention of blood pressure was almost a taboo; it was not something that polite people asked their doctors about. But it is information you have a right and a need to know. You know your weight, height, and age; your blood pressure should be included among your vital statistics as well. You should have your blood pressure checked every time you see a doctor—any doctor! Hypertension is often initially discovered during a routine check, and many find out about their condition when they buy insurance.

Unfortunately, blood pressure is often a neglected determination. In a recent study of hospital charts, about 25 percent of the patients had not had their blood pressure taken by the doctor. In a study in Virginia only 20 percent of doctors in subspecialties routinely checked a patient's blood pressure. When a patient had been found to have high blood pressure during a screening and was referred to his own doctor, nearly one-third received no treatment at all. Some of these patients were not even given a return appointment! Consider the case of Harold.

Harold was a dynamo of a salesman; he got his work done quickly and expected no less from his subordinates. He had more vitality than most men of forty-five. That is why he was especially puzzled when he began to grow more fatigued in the midafternoons of long business days. That had never happened to him before. His work did not suffer, because he forced himself to even greater effort. However, the people around him noticed a personality change; he was irritable at home and demanding at work. But there was nobody who could keep up with him in sales, and when an opening appeared in management, Harold was the unanimous choice. The promotion meant a higher salary. His wife quickly translated that into a larger home, and the real estate agent convinced him he needed a larger mortgage. The bank prudently insisted on his increasing his life insurance to cover the difference. After the insurance physical, the doctor told Harold that he had high blood pressure. Harold procrastinated for several years before having his pressure rechecked. Harold eventually came under treatment, and his pressure fell from 180/110 to a more livable 125/85; his fatigue disappeared, and he was easier to live with. Harold's symptoms were only meaningful to him in retrospect. He would not have sought medical attention on his own.

As noted, our blood pressure varies daily according to our needs. It should be normal when we are at rest, but we are not always resting. A special device has been fabricated that continuously measures the blood pressure and records it. In one experiment, the wearer was to keep the machine with him all day, writing down what he did and when he did it. Later, the blood pressure recording for the entire twenty-four hours could be analyzed. A young doctor agreed to be the guinea pig for the study. He was advised to behave in his usual fashion and to disregard the device. His initial blood pressure was normal. However, when the young doctor became bored while listening to his professor talk, his pressure dropped to very low levels. He went home after work and fought with his wife, and his blood pressure shot up promptly. The rise was temporary, and he later made up with her. Their reconciliation must have been complete, because later that night they had intercourse and his blood pressure rose dramatically. Finally, it drifted down to its lowest level, when he fell into a deep sleep.

The important point to realize is that there were moments during the day when the doctor's blood pressure was high, but he did not have high blood pressure. The elevations were all related to appropriate situations, and they were all transient. Even someone with high blood pressure may drift down to normal if he or she is in a deep sleep. The average blood pressure while the patient is quiet and awake is the determinant of whether high blood pressure is present. By taking multiple readings, a temporary rise can be properly recognized. I often teach my patients with hypertension to take their own pressure, to assure better control. Home readings can avoid the anxiety associated with a doctor's office and help regulate the amount of medication required. The procedure is painless, inexpensive, and accurate. Some authorities feel—although perhaps they are exaggerating—that the blood-pressure apparatus is a more important medical instrument for the home than a thermometer for people over forty-five.

Treatment of high blood pressure requires a lifelong commitment. What happens if you just forget the whole thing? Basically, you either suffer complications or you do not. There are many complications, and they are all unpleasant.

The most important complication is an acceleration of the process of atherosclerosis. High blood pressure may encourage the filtration of more cholesterol through the arterial wall, may injure the wall by the mechanical strain of the increased pressure, or may stimulate the mutation of smooth muscle cells in the intima and thereby cause the development of new plaque. It may do all these things; it may do none of them. We do not know why high blood pressure accelerates atherosclerosis. We know that it does.

With the increase in atherosclerosis comes an increased risk of strokes, the destruction of part of the brain due to interference with its blood supply. When a stroke occurs, the patient may lose partial control over half his body. About 1/4 million people suffer a stroke every year. For them a stroke means a dramatic change from independence and concern about the day-to-day minutiae, to being disabled, dependent, and defeated. Many people with high blood pressure who experience a stroke will be unable ever again to speak, read, walk, or care for their personal hygiene.

Nor is the dramatic disaster of a stroke the only way that high blood pressure affects the brain. There can be minor losses of the brain's functional ability over a long period, where the patient in the final stages becomes demented or incoherent. The brain loses some of its sharpness, and yet no single causative event can be identified. A study followed a group of elderly patients for ten years: those who had normal blood pressure retained their intelligence; those with high blood pressure had measurable losses.

High blood pressure may also cause heart failure because of the extra work the heart has to perform to overcome the high pressure in the arterial system. The heart is stretched, the kidneys begin to retain salt and water, and the lungs become congested. The patient experiences cough, shortness of breath, and swollen ankles. The heart can no longer keep up with the demands of the body, and fatigue becomes a relentless companion. Luckily, heart failure due to high blood pressure can be avoided by proper control of the blood pressure. The following story concerns a patient of mine whose history is typical of many hypertensive people.

Helene was a fifty-seven-year-old clerk. For many years she had an elevated blood pressure but had no symptoms. She was active and vivacious. Then Helene noted that she was still tired after a good night's sleep. She developed a cough and subsequently shortness of breath. Her shoes did not fit as well as they once had, and she discovered that she needed the next larger size to be comfortable. She was suffering heart failure, with a blood pressure of 185/98, when I examined her. Helene required hospitalization and extensive treatment, but she recovered. Her blood pressure was controlled, and she was again able to resume her employment and usual activities.

Hypertension also affects the kidneys and can lead to kidney failure. Since kidney disease can lead to high blood pressure, a vicious circle can be established in the body. High blood pressure can also cause hemorrhages to appear in the visual lining of the eye. These may heal, but there will be a partial loss of sight.

At one time the two most powerful men in the world both suffered from the same disease, which finally disabled and killed them. Franklin

Roosevelt and Joseph Stalin both had high blood pressure, and they died of its complications. Despite Stalin's paranoia, it was not a plot but the simple lack of an effective drug that doomed him. Roosevelt received a sedative but no real antihypertensive. Anyone reading this book can and should receive far better treatment if hypertension is discovered.

There is more that you should know about the diagnosis and treatment of high blood pressure. Remember, the more you know, the better you will cooperate with treatment, and the less likely you will be to suffer the consequences of hypertension. Good treatment requires a close working partnership between you and your doctor. The physician must perform a careful and complete physical examination in order to deal with your high blood pressure intelligently. It helps him identify any complications, either present or potential. An important part of the examination is a careful look at the inner lining (retina) of the eyes. By shining an intense light in your eyes the doctor can observe the blood vessels in their native state. The earliest signs of hypertension can be recognized when the arteries in the retina begin to compress the veins beneath them and cause little nicks. Later signs include areas of hemorrhage and swellings.

We can identify the actual cause of high blood pressure in a small percentage of hypertensives. These cases are all potentially reversible; theoretically, if we identify and remove the cause, the hypertension should disappear. Sometimes it does, but not always. The known causes require considerable medical detective work to uncover. Some clues can be recognized by a layperson. This kind of self-examination can provide a clue to a curable hypertension and potentially save a life. Remember, the vast majority of hypertensives can be treated even if we do not know the cause of the hypertension.

The first rare but curable type of high blood pressure is called coarctation of the aorta. You are either born with it or escape entirely; it does not develop in later life. The disease is caused by a distinct narrowing or pinching in the aorta, which occurs below the point where the arteries to the brain and upper limbs branch off. Since the narrowing greatly increases resistance to blood flow, the blood pressure in the arms and head is higher, but the legs receive much less blood and have a lower pressure. Coarctation may be suspected when the doctor feels no pulse in the groin. Almost everyone can feel his own normal pulse there, especially if he lies down and gently compresses the midportion of the groin where the leg and torso meet. Another way of checking is to take the blood pressure in the leg as well as in the arm. In healthy people the blood pressure in the leg is higher than in the arm. Once the diagnosis is made, the condition can be repaired surgically with excellent long-term results.

Another type of curable hypertension, called pheochromacytoma, is caused by a tumor on the adrenal glands. The normal adrenal glands sit on top of the kidneys. Their function is to secrete adrenaline, which elevates the blood pressure and makes the heart beat faster when we are excited or threatened by an external danger. This is the so-called fight-or-flight response, which may have helped our primitive ancestors to escape dangerous situations. The response is less necessary in today's world, but we keep calling it up in times of anxiety or stress. Most people quickly resume their tranquil state after an exciting event, and the blood pressure drifts down to normal. In rare instances a tumor (pheochromocytoma) develops in one of the adrenal glands and releases large amounts of adrenaline or the related chemical norepinephrine.

The patient with such a tumor may have persistent or intermittent hypertension, depending on the secretion of the tumor. Other symptoms—headaches, palpitations, nausea, fainting, nervousness—can occur in attacks and help in the recognition of this rare form of hypertension. In some patients, attacks can be brought on by the patient or by the doctor's merely massaging the abdomen. The blood pressure during these episodes can reach alarming levels and, if left uncorrected or undiagnosed, can lead to a stroke. The pheochromocytoma can be diagnosed by finding by-products of adrenaline in the urine. Once diagnosed, surgical removal of the tumor will usually resolve the problem and the patient will regain normal blood pressure.

Another form of curable hypertension is caused by an adrenal tumor that produces excess amounts of a hormone called aldosterone. This hormone causes the loss of potassium and the retention of sodium. The loss of potassium may result in weakness, numbness, and an increased volume of urination. Retention of sodium causes excessive salt and water in the body and a rise in blood pressure. This type of adrenal tumor can be removed and a cure effected.

Still another form of hypertension related to the adrenal glands is caused by the secretion of other adrenal hormones, related to cortisone, that raise the blood pressure. The victims of this disease named Cushing's syndrome often are obese women with purple stretch marks of the abdomen and a small "buffalo hump" of fatty tissue between the shoulder blades just below the neck. Their faces are round, almost moonlike in appearance, and they have a form of acne that is unusual in adults. Cushing's syndrome is not always caused by a tumor. Sometimes the glands just enlarge and begin to secrete too much hormone without any change in the glands' normal architecture. It is as though they had received a defective message to increase production when the body had no additional need. Surgery and a variety of drugs may help these patients.

The kidneys are another more frequent source of curable hypertension. The original experiments to cause high blood pressure in laboratory animals involved the use of a clamp that gradually occluded the blood flow to the kidneys. A comparable mechanism functions in some people who develop a critical narrowing of one or both of the arteries to the kidneys. This deprivation of blood flow results in increased kidney production of the hormone renin. Renin then acts on another chemical in the blood (angiotensin) and produces the most powerful blood-pressure-elevating chemical known to exist. Renin also increases the secretion of aldosterone, which causes more salt retention and further blood-pressure elevation.

The narrowing in the kidneys' arteries can be muscular, especially in the young, or a manifestation of atherosclerosis, as we noted earlier. The type of obstruction and the age of the patient are strong influences on the likelihood of successful surgery; the younger person with a nonatherosclerotic occlusion is more likely to benefit than the older patient with an extensive atherosclerotic lesion. Even after surgery not everyone is cured, and a significant number must continue to take antihypertensive medication.

There is a rare and easily curable type of high blood pressure that most people will not believe exists: it is possible to get hypertension from eating too much licorice. For these few susceptible people the cure is simple—kick the licorice habit. Another unusual form of curable high blood pressure that we have previously mentioned is found in young women who take the birth-control pill; the hypertension will usually regress if the pill is discontinued. In both these forms of curable hypertension, the diagnosis can be made by the patient.

Since we know some of the factors that control the blood pressure, we can select methods of reducing it. The first class of antihypertension medicines is called diuretics; they increase urine flow. Diuretics act to reduce the amount of salt and water in the circulating blood, and therefore they lower the amount of blood the heart pumps out. There are a large number of diuretics available, but when used correctly they all have about the same total effect on blood pressure. Most of the diuretics cause a loss of potassium as well as sodium, although a few cause a retention of potassium; these can be used in combination with the potassium-losing diuretics in order to avoid dangerously low levels of potassium. The diuretics are usually the first drug a physician prescribes in treating a mild hypertensive. They are reasonably effective and have an additional advantage of potentiating the action of other nondiuretic antihypertensive drugs, many of which cause the retention of salt. Their ease of administration and low cost are additional advantages.

Unfortunately, although the diuretics are relatively safe, they can, and do, cause a variety of side effects. Some diuretics such as chlorthiazide (known also under several trade names, including Diuril) can cause the formation of kidney stones because they raise the uric-acid level in the blood. This same rise in blood uric acid can cause a painful episode of gout. Diuretics can also cause a rise in blood sugar and interfere with the control of diabetes. Like almost every drug ever synthesized, diuretics produce some allergic reactions, which usually include rash and fever.

One of the older drugs that has been used for high blood pressure is reserpine (trade name Serpasil). Reserpine also causes relaxation and a distinct slowing of the heart. It was originally used as a crude extract of a root found in India, where it had been known as a tranquilizing drug long before the development of modern pharmacology. The drug enjoyed wide usage in the United States when first released because it was mildly effective and because there were not many other useful drugs for the purpose. As reports accumulated about the side effects of the drug—severe depression, nightmares, and weight gain—and newer drugs became available, reserpine was less widely used.

A second class of drugs useful for the management of hypertension is the so-called beta blockers. These drugs work by blocking the effects of stimulation of the nervous system. They cause the heartbeat to be slower and less powerful. The heart does less work and the amount of blood pumped out falls, as does the blood pressure. Beta blockers can also free an angina patient from pain. They are especially useful in the common situation where coronary heart disease and hypertension coexist. At the present time, only one beta blocker is available in the United States: it is named propranolol (trade name Inderal). I have been recently involved in research on another beta blocker called Timilol, which will be available in the future. Side effects caused by propranolol appear to be infrequent, but it can intensify asthma or congestive heart failure if given to patients with these problems.

The third category of drugs used in hypertension is the vasodilators. They work by dilating the arterioles, which are the sites of the resistance of blood flow, thereby lowering the blood pressure. The first available dilator was hydralazine (Apresoline). Hydralazine enjoyed a brief period of popularity when it was first released, as all new drugs do. Unfortunately, it also speeds the heart rate, which tends to balance the drop in blood pressure caused by the lowering of resistance. Hydralazine also causes chest pain, palpitations, a peculiar rash resembling that of a connective-tissue disease known as lupus, and inflammation of the lining around the heart and the lungs. These side effects can be avoided by careful adjustment of the dose. Physicians often combine the use of hydralazine, which acts to dilate the arteries, with propranolol, which slows the heart. The combination is more effective than either component, and smaller doses of both drugs can be used so that side effects are infrequent.

A new dilator has recently been released for use. It is called prazosin (Minipres). I had the opportunity to be one of the investigators who studied the drug before it was approved by the Food and Drug Administration. Prazosin can be used in mild hypertension. Unfortunately, in some patients it causes dizziness, drowsiness, palpitations, weakness, and—in 1 percent of those who take it—sudden loss of consciousness.

Some antihypertensive drugs interfere with the nervous control of the resistance at the arterioles. During stress, exercise, or emotion, a message is sent by the nervous system to the muscles in the arterioles causing them to contract; resistance is increased, and the blood pressure goes up. Drugs that prevent this progression help reduce hypertension.

The most potent drug that interferes with the nervous-system message to raise the blood pressure is called guanethidine (Ismelin). It can be used in more severe forms of hypertension and preferentially lowers the standing blood pressure. That is the catch: it works best to prevent an increase in resistance when you stand. The erect posture forces blood to pool in the legs. By increasing resistance in the blood vessels in the legs, we all normally force blood to circulate to other, more necessary, parts of the body. Guanethidine prevents that fine adjustment, and the blood pools in the legs on standing. That means that there is not enough blood circulating in the brain; the patient may get dizzy or faint. That is not the only thing that guanethidine does. It interferes with male ejaculation, so that though a man may remain potent and carry out the sex act, he cannot culminate it.

A newer antihypertensive drug is alpha-methyl dopa (Aldomet), which works in a unique fashion. It resembles norepinephrine, which acts as a message transmitter at the nerve endings. Alpha-methyl dopa interferes with the normal messages sent to raise the blood pressure and so lowers the pressure. It is useful for patients with severe hypertension, and most patients can take it without any side effects. However, it can cause an anemia as the result of destruction of the red blood cells and may produce impairment in liver function. It also causes sedation, nasal stuffiness, and slowing of the heart. In men it can even result in breast enlargement and impotence.

What emerges from this brief survey of the more commonly used antihypertensive drugs is that they can all cause a variety of interesting and unpleasant side effects. That is the crux of the problem. The treated patient with high blood pressure may have more discomfort than his untreated counterpart, who is usually asymptomatic until a disaster such as a heart attack or stroke occurs. To maintain control requires good motivation by the patient and careful use of appropriate drugs by the physician. With patience and cooperation, an antihypertensive program that is effective without causing intolerable side effects can be achieved by most patients.

CHAPTER EIGHT

Exercise and Coronary-Artery Disease

We are all animals. We are part of the animal kingdom, and we take on certain characteristics of this group; we require regular physical activity. Today some people are so sedentary that they may be easily confused with plants or sculpture. Good health rewards us with a sense of vitality and freedom from illness, but we must work at maintaining this state. Part of the price is regular physical activity.

Only in recent years have we had to consider exercise as supplemental. Consider the situation of our forefathers. Their daily chores provided all the exercise their muscles needed. Most transportation was by foot, manufacturing jobs generally required heavy physical effort, and household duties demanded strenuous work. With the onset of the industrial revolution and "progress," there were many changes in the way things were done. Machines began to replace the individual's muscle power, and the wide use of cheap energy supplanted personal physical effort for almost everything.

Machines and cheap energy also permitted a quantum increase in the manufactured goods available. The enrichment of life was widespread and still continues. But as a nation we became more sedentary and less physically fit, and the incidence of coronary atherosclerosis rose. Thus, the reduction in daily exercise had far-reaching consequences that were not anticipated.

Let us briefly examine the physiology of exercise. We all need oxygen to sustain our lives. Oxygen combines with a foodstuff fuel, usually the sugar in the cells, to provide energy the body needs. If a cell is deprived of oxygen long enough, it will die. Air and oxygen are moved into our lungs as we breathe, and the oxygen is absorbed into the bloodstream. The blood is distributed throughout the body, preferentially to areas of greatest need. Exercise makes more and more demands on our muscles, which require a gradually increasing supply of oxygen, and therefore of blood. However, there is a point at which the heart cannot supply any further increment of blood. The muscles begin to burn fuel without available oxygen, and a by-product called lactic acid is formed. Finally, despite all the motivation in the world, fatigue becomes overwhelming and the exercise must be discontinued. The amount of oxygen that can be used at this maximal effort is a good measure of the individual's ability to perform. In trained athletes the "maximum oxygen utilization measurement" is high; in those who do not exercise consistently, it is low. The measurement can be improved by regular exercise.

The normal heart has a maximum rate, which helps determine exactly what a person can do. No amount of effort or desire will coax the normal heart to beat any faster. We can now predict the maximum heart rate even before we stress the individual, by subtracting the person's age from 220 beats per minute. This means that a fifty-year-old person can reach a maximum heart rate of 220 minus 50, or 170. Depending on physical condition, a person must achieve at least 60 percent of the maximum heart rate in order to obtain the benefits of exercise.

What are the benefits of exercise? In general, one feels and looks good. The muscles have more tone and strength; the joints and ligaments are more supple; one has greater agility and coordination. Fatigue and physical stress are tolerated better. A regular exercise program keeps a person trim and helps burn up excess calories. The skin becomes more flexible and the face looks alive. There is an improved sense of body image. Exercise is an excellent way to work off tension and can be considered a natural tranquilizer.

These are all worthwhile objectives, but the hidden benefits of exercise are equally important. Exercise increases the heart's pumping ability—which, after all, is its primary function. The heart rate, both at rest and during exercise, becomes slower because there is an increase in the amount of blood the heart expels with each contraction. The pressure usually rises during active exercise, but it will be lower at rest than originally. In fact, blood pressure often improves after a regular exercise program. Exercise also encourages the growth of new, auxiliary channels between the coronary arteries that help to nourish the heart, especially if there is narrowing caused by atherosclerosis. Although the evidence in humans is not conclusive, animals forced to exercise regularly show a richer network of these auxiliary channels than animals that are not exercised.

Exercise can help lower the cholesterol and triglyceride levels in the blood. In a recent finding, long-distance runners, who have a much smaller chance of heart attack, showed more high-density lipoprotein in the blood than inactive normals. Exercise may contribute to the increase of this lipoprotein, but in what way is not known. What is known is that the high-density lipoprotein acts to transport cholesterol from tissue sites (including the arteries) to the liver, where it can be degraded and eliminated. Thus, there may be some connection between the presence of high-density lipoprotein in the blood and a lower rate of heart attacks. The minimal level of exercise required to raise the blood level of the high-density lipoprotein is uncertain, but the runners studied were running at least fifteen miles a week.

The kinds of exercise most beneficial to maintaining good health are basically those that require the use of large masses of muscle. The exercise you personally select should be enjoyable and easily accessible. The best resolution is worthless if you choose to swim out of doors daily and live in northern Maine. For most people, the best single exercise is walking briskly. Walking is cheap, available, and lends itself to quantification. Other acceptable alternatives, depending on climate, include jogging, swimming, bicycling, ice skating, skiing, canoeing, tennis, golf, and volleyball.

Pick an activity that you can do repetitively. Team sports have limitations. Joining an organization interested in a particular sport will help sustain your commitment and provide other personal advantages. A local Y may have exercise classes and organized running programs; these will add some social exposure to your exercises. If you walk, jog, or run, a simple pedometer will help you keep track of your progress and encourage you to continue. The important thing is to sustain your motivation. Daily additions to your total exercise program can include walking the stairs instead of using the elevator, walking between appointments, and parking as far as is practical from your work site.

People who become interested in maintaining physical fitness frequently ask how often they must work out. There are some guidelines. First, determine what you are trying to do. If you are under thirty, not overweight, and have no risk factors associated with heart disease, you will probably benefit from as few as two sessions a week. But if you are over thirty and have a weight problem or another significant risk factor, then three or more sessions a week are desirable. The duration of the exercise depends on the intensity. Singles tennis is more demanding than doubles. Cross-country skiing takes more energy in very cold weather. There seems to be a myth that exercise must result in muscle discomfort in order to be of value. If you experience muscle aches and pains, excessive fatigue, or sleeplessness after a workout, you may have overdone it. It is preferable to arrange brief sessions if you are just starting and have been physically inactive. Plan on doing less than you think you can initially, and very gradually increase the duration until each session is at least thirty minutes long.

Duration is the critical word. In running, the important thing is how long you continue rather than how fast you go. If you want to increase your endurance, you need not compete to win medals. For most people interested in fitness, the best approach is to experiment gradually to find the proper niche.

Here are some basic suggestions that will be useful to the beginner. Warm up gradually. Do not apply your peak power immediately. If you are running and do not enjoy calisthenics, go slowly the first few hundred yards. After exercising, walk around after your peak effort and then wait a few moments before you jump into a hot shower. If you forget these warnings you may become dizzy or even faint, because blood will pool in your legs and not enough will reach your brain.

The best investment anyone can make before starting an exercise program is to get the proper shoes. Comfortable, well-fitting shoes will prevent injuries and will make your workout much more pleasant. Newer developments in jogging shoes have made your old pair of sneakers obsolete. Although you can run or walk in any kind of clothing, if you intend to stick with the activity, you might regard a running suit an inexpensive investment that will pay for itself. A word of caution here: vinyl or plastic sweat suits are potentially dangerous and should be avoided. Enthusiasts who recommend them feel that they encourage sweating and thereby weight loss, but this is foolish. You will sweat enough from the exercise. Any weight loss caused by perspiring is promptly and completely regained by your next drink.

Another good suggestion before starting an exercise program is to have a complete physical examination. If you are over forty and have risk factors, your doctor may suggest an exercise stress test, in which your electrocardiogram is recorded while you run on a treadmill. The initial physical examination should always include a resting electrocardiogram and blood tests for cholesterol, triglycerides, and sugar.

It may be interesting to review some of the studies that have shown the increased risk of coronary heart disease that accompanies the sedentary life-style. A group at the Harvard Medical School in the 1950s examined the differences between sets of Irish brothers who met certain rigid criteria. In each set there was no more than a five-year age difference, and at least ten years of observations were available. One brother of each pair had emigrated to Boston and one had remained in Ireland. The brothers in Ireland were physically more active and traveled largely by foot and bicycle; their American counterparts drove cars. The physicians found that there was a much higher incidence of heart disease in the brothers who lived in Boston. This difference was attributed to the difference in activity.

Another study examined railroad clerks who were much less active than their coworkers who were switchmen. The switchmen were much less likely to suffer from coronary-artery disease. Still another study focused on people who lived on a single kibbutz in Israel. They shared the same food, living accommodations, and stresses. They had a variety of tasks, some sedentary and others physically active. The incidence of heart disease was higher among the sedentary workers.

The British double-decker buses contain a driver who sits and steers the bus and a conductor who collects fares, going up and down the stairs many times a day. The conductors are much less likely to develop heart attacks than the drivers. Here again physical activity appears protective.

When Midwestern farmers were compared with their sedentary city counterparts, the farmers were found to suffer far fewer heart attacks. Postal workers were also compared. Clerks were far less active than mailmen, who walked their respective routes every working day, often carrying heavy sacks of mail. The mailmen had fewer heart attacks.

Another report concerns the Masai tribe of Africa, in which the men walk with their cattle, averaging over ten miles a day. The coronary arteries of those who died natural deaths were examined; they were found to be large and free of atherosclerotic narrowing.

All these studies have some defects, but the mainstream connection is clear. When people are physically active throughout their adult lives, they are much less likely to develop coronary heart disease.

The Tarahumara Indians of northern Mexico are a good example. They live in a rugged, inhospitable area with little tillable land. In order to survive, they have adjusted well to their environment and can trace their ancestors back almost two thousand years. The name *Tarahumara* literally means "foot runner." Running is their recreation and a determinant of social position. It also represents a way of hunting for food. Incredible as it may sound, the Tarahumara hunt deer and turkey by running after them for days at a time until the animal drops from exhaustion. Despite this, the Tarahumara diet consists largely of corn, beans, and vegetables; they eat very little meat. Their daily intake of cholesterol is low.

The major source of recreation among the Tarahumara is a type of kickball game that has been modified over the years into a race covering more than seventy-five miles. The men run over rough trails kicking a wooden ball, continuing day and night until someone crosses the winning line. The women also compete in their own running events, and children are encouraged to run as soon as they have mastered walking.

The Tarahumara are poor and have very little in the way of capital goods; many are undernourished. An average Tarahumara adult male has a cholesterol level of 100 mg.%, which is less than half the ideal level and far less than the American adult average of 235 mg.%. Something else the Tarahumara do not have is heart disease or heart attacks.

Although it may not be possible for the reader to adopt the Tarahumara life-style, an increase in exercise and reduction of meat intake are achievable goals. So is the reduction of the risk of coronary atherosclerosis.

In the last ten years there has been a dramatic shift in medical opinion. Not too many years ago the patient who recovered from a heart attack was told only what *not* to do. Now there are many cardiac rehabilitation centers that encourage and monitor graded and increasing exercise. The physician can write an exercise prescription, and the patient is able to increase his effort gradually while under expert observation. Some of these programs have taken patients after recovery from a heart attack and converted them to successful marathon runners (the marathon is more than twenty-six miles). There is an apparent reduction in the annual death rate among those who have successfully continued in a rehabilitation exercise program. Not all authorities agree on the value of specific exercise programs, but the early reports are optimistic.

The role of exercise in health and disease is still under intense investigation and discussion. There are zealots with opposite views. Until the muddy waters of controversy clear there are several guidelines that can be useful. Build an exercise program into your day-to-day life. Have a competent physician examine you before you engage in any competitive or vigorous exercise. Start at a low level of effort that is easy for you to complete. Gradually increase the duration and/or frequency of your efforts. Learn the pleasure of working up a good sweat. After a while you will find that the activity becomes more meaningful to you and, like virtue, becomes its own reward. Don't get discouraged by your lack of Olympic talent. You should be in an exercise program to help your body and your mind reach their fullest potential. If you are persistent you'll soon find that the secondary gains you achieve make the effort and time commitment worthwhile.

CHAPTER NINE

Overweight and Dieting

Most people probably agree that being fat is undesirable; at the very least, most fashionable clothes are designed for, and modeled by, the slim. More important, extra pounds mean that it is harder to climb a flight of stairs, run for a bus, or keep cool in hot weather. As if these penalties were not enough, fat people live shorter lives on the average and have more chronic and disabling diseases.

A frequently heard description of a heavy person is "jolly"; actually, many fat people are secretly depressed. Well-adjusted heavyweights have in many cases tried a variety of diets and fads and have abandoned the struggle. Inside most fat people a thin person is desperately trying to break out. Although buttons and posters claim that "fat is beautiful," I personally do not believe it and neither, I think, do the majority of those afflicted.

A study involving 3,983 pilots in training for the Royal Canadian Air Force during World War II has provided valuable information on the role of excess weight in the development of coronary atherosclerosis. The men were followed carefully during the twenty-six years after their training period, and 390 of them developed coronary-artery disease. Analysis of the data showed that those who were overweight carried a greater risk of heart attack and sudden death. This relationship was most marked in men under forty and did not become evident until the men had been followed for sixteen years. The relationship persisted even after the effects of age and high blood pressure had been taken into consideration.

Obesity is associated with a variety of risk factors, including high blood pressure and elevation of the blood sugar, cholesterol, and triglyceride levels. All these factors interact and result in an increased risk of disability, disease, and death. Compared with the average population, the obese suffer more heart attacks, strokes, kidney diseases, liver and gall bladder malignancies, diabetes mellitus, cirrhosis of the liver, and arthritis. They are more likely to die during minor operations, such as hernia or intestinal surgery. The obese must do more work when they breathe, and they become short of breath more easily. Excess weight also imposes an increased work load on the heart, even if it is free of structural diseases such as coronary atherosclerosis. Roughly thirty pounds of excess weight will reduce life expectancy by four years.

One factor that contributes to obesity is the increased variety of foods available because of the development of refrigeration. In colonial America people could not store milk, butter, ice cream, or fresh meat in large quantities. This forced them to be more dependent on fruits, vegetables, and grains. Most foods were prepared at home, and there was much less consumption of sugar. Additives were unnecessary, and only rarely were preprocessed foods used. The diet contained less fat and more roughage.

Primitive humans led a feast-or-famine existence. Food supplies were not always assured. A strong appetite provided motivation to hunt and gather edibles. Those who hunted well survived longer. Those who survived longer had better opportunities to reproduce; so we evolved with a very strong, well-developed appetite. But when humans drew together to form societies and began to produce an overabundance of food, the survival advantage of a sharp appetite disappeared. Adults today have to make a conscious effort to avoid becoming overweight. Where once a few extra pounds were a sign of prosperity, they have become a liability.

Americans have developed the most efficient agricultural and food-distribution industries in the world. This means that they can spend proportionately less of their earned income on food than can any other society. It also means that they eat an excess of meat from animals that have been force-fed to make their meat tender, marbled with fat, and high in cholesterol. We have a national sweet tooth that consumes a hundred pounds of sweetening a year per person. Junk foods and empty calories are made attractive to our children through a frighteningly efficient system of advertising. Vitamins and purified proteins are suggested as panaceas by self-appointed experts. There is no need for purified protein as a supplement; a balanced diet provides all the protein and other nutrients we require. There are plenty of naturally available vitamins and minerals in fruits, vegetables, and cereals. We need only the knowledge to choose wisely from the cornucopia of available foodstuffs.

Eating has become more than a way to assuage our hunger. We use eating as a form of social intercourse. Many of us expect to be offered something to eat or drink during business meetings. In childhood we are urged to clean our plates, and if served food is not consumed, many consider it sinful.

It takes about 3,500 calories to equal a pound of body flesh. If you add or lose a pound, then 3,500 calories are consumed or utilized. The average adult needs about 15 calories per pound per day to maintain body weight. One can lose weight only by eating less than is burned on a long-range basis. For example, a man weighing 150 pounds must consume 2,250 calories a day to maintain his weight. If he consumed 1,750 calories, he would lose 500 calories each day. Assuming that he does this for a week, he will burn 3,500 calories more than he eats and will weigh one pound less. These are all approximate figures, and that is where many would-be dieters go wrong.

By far the most important reason for gradual weight gain in middle age is the lack of enough exercise. In earlier eras the preparation of food was a daily physical chore, and shopping meant a walk rather than a car ride. Even if there were occasions when excess food was eaten, the opportunity to burn it off was always present. People spent long hours working with their muscles; it was easier to balance the supply and demand of calories.

The changes since those days have been remarkable. Progress has extracted a price, however. Along with the greater availability of all sorts of foods has come a reduction of the energy cost of moving around. The average home is increasingly mechanized. Few dieters clean their clothes by hand. In many bathrooms we could find such calorie-saving devices as an automatic electric toothbrush. What one puts into the body is no longer balanced by the output of muscle power; consequently, the excess calories are stored as fat.

Life in underdeveloped countries today can be compared in many ways with early American life. People work with their muscles, and walking is the method of travel; fewer adults are obese. What we do through mechanization is still carried out by hand. A well may supply the needed water only after hand pumping, and one must heat water over a fire whose fuel is hand gathered. The less fortunate nations may have a lower standard of living, but they have a lower death rate from coronary atherosclerosis. It is almost as if a capricious natural force was balancing the pros and cons of progress and civilization.

Another factor in addition to lack of exercise explains the gradual weight gain that comes with increasing years. As you age, the body burns fewer calories during usual activities. You may need fifty fewer calories a day than you did several years ago. However, the way you eat is primarily determined by habit and social mores, so you tend to maintain a constant diet even though you have a declining energy need. The result is that you get heavier as you age, even if you eat no more than when you were younger.

The body contains, in addition to flesh, fluids that are in a state of flux. If you go on a crash diet and lose ten pounds in two days, the chances are that nine pounds are water. There are also several fad diets recently promulgated that suggest fasting as a means of losing weight. This is certainly effective; famines and concentration camps have demonstrated that well enough. But fasting may be unsafe and become more difficult as one goes along, and weight losses will probably prove impermanent. Why does it become more difficult? The body in its wisdom recognizes the onset of starvation. The longer you fast, the slower your metabolism becomes; eventually, you have to deny yourself five thousand calories to lose a single pound.

Insurance companies know that a higher death rate accompanies excess weight and that the increased mortality is not limited to cardiovascular diseases. Remember that insurance companies are in business to make money; the longer you live, the more money they make. If you are fat, they charge you more money to insure your life. They are wagering that you will die earlier, that they will have to pay claims earlier, and that they will therefore make less money from the premiums. Mortality rises in rough proportion to the degree of overweight; the more obese you are, the higher the risk of death at an early age.

How can you tell if you are overweight? Most people know deep down inside if they have put on some weight; a few truly are uncertain. Unless you are a weight lifter or a professional football player, the standard height and weight charts are adequate. (Charts do not separate muscle mass from fat.) A glance at your naked figure in a mirror will probably reveal whether you are dealing with fat or muscle. Another way to tell is to pinch the flesh around your waist. If there is more than an inch between your fingers, you have failed the pinch test. Your waist measurement, if you are a man, probably should never exceed thirty-four inches, so your belt size tells you if you are overweight. Weight should not increase once you reach your early twenties; if it has, you probably can do without it.

Once you have decided that you are overweight and that you want to reduce, you must go about it sensibly. You want to achieve and maintain your ideal weight. That automatically excludes fad or crash diets. Most people who say they want to lose weight fast have not decided that they want to keep the weight off. They have too much fun going up and down. If you lose weight too fast, you will gain it back just as rapidly.

During several years of research I have developed a cereal-based diet that will help you lose weight and keep it off. It will, in addition, lower the cholesterol and triglyceride levels in the blood. The diet is balanced and nutritious and consists of familiar day-to-day foods. Meals are limited in meats, fish, chicken, cheeses, and eggs and provide many more cereal servings than you would expect on a reducing diet. The fats used are largely polyunsaturated vegetable oils. The diet is inexpensive to follow and succeeds without deceptive water shifts. Success is assured if you are conscientious; in fact, twenty-five of twenty-six volunteers lost weight on it. The diet appears in detail in Appendix 1.

Just as it is important to know what you are eating when you choose to diet, it is important to know about the popular fallacies concerning dieting. The most persistent myth is that the glands are somehow responsible for your weight gain. That is almost never correct. The notion is encouraged by some popular diet books that suggest that weight gain is caused by a factor you cannot control and so relieves you of any responsibility. Although it is not necessary to carry a sense of guilt about obesity, there is no sense in relying on make-believe, either. Thyroid disorders do not account for any significant number of the fat people you know.

Another recent "non-diagnosis fad" is the frequency of hypoglycemia, or low blood sugar, among overweight people. Although there are individuals with a low blood sugar after they have fasted, most of them are thin—not fat—and many have no symptoms. If you wish to blame hypoglycemia for your eating and weight problems, you may be misleading yourself.

Some people really believe that only certain foods such as bread or spaghetti make them fat and that they can eat meat or fat with impunity. Unfortunately, a calorie is a measure of heat energy and not a demon in which you can choose to disbelieve. If you eat more than you burn, you will gain weight and vice versa. It is the total caloric, or energy, value of the food you eat that determines your weight. Everyone who eats fewer calories than the body uses must lose weight!

The blossoming of a variety of low- or no-carbohydrate diets is another pernicious recent craze. Low-carbohydrate diets are usually high in fat, cholesterol, and calories. Despite many claims, little has appeared in the scientific literature that demonstrates a real advantage of such diets over a long period of time. For the impatient pseudodieter they offer the mirage of rapid weight loss, because such diets cause the body initially to lose water. Soon the water is replaced, the weight returns, and the patient is still obese. Quickie diets such as this often produce uncomfortable symptoms and may be nutritionally deficient.

The so-called one-food diets—for instance, the grapefruit diet and the egg diet—are also unbalanced and represent poor nutrition. They have a fad value for those who demand the latest gimmick. Only after you decide to be thin for life with good nutrition can you hope to succeed.

Another fake diet that everyone has tried at least once is the technique of skipping meals. The usual scenario runs thus: Having gorged himself the night before, the dieter awakens with no appetite and resolutely decides to skip breakfast. By eleven o'clock there is a coffee break, and with the black coffee a Danish pastry disappears, on the assumption that it is almost lunch time. A lunch of salad and more black coffee satisfies the need for self-flagellation. By supper time the dieter feels quite virtuous—and hungry. He has a "regular" supper— which is a euphemism for a fourteen-ounce steak (which contains more than a thousand calories), coffee, and dessert (probably another four hundred calories). That night, about two hours after supper, he is in the refrigerator again, and by the time he goes to bed, he has had the equivalent of a second supper by munching on cheese, crackers, a chicken leg, and some leftover pie. This phenomenon was described by Dr. Albert Stunkard of New York in a well-regarded 1959 medical article as the night-eating syndrome. Despite skipping breakfast and eating nothing caloric for lunch, the "dieter" has put in thirty-six hundred calories and not lost any weight. It is a far better technique to eat three balanced meals a day, plan on a specific snack every night, and use a diet that is sensible enough to stick with over the long haul.

Another false path is the diet-pill approach. After millions of doses and hundreds of research studies, the facts are these: The pills help only a few people and then only for about two weeks. There is no pill that can convert an obese person to a thin one. There are side effects reported for every pill available. In short, the pills are not worthwhile; dieting is. Some people do manage to lose weight on a diet pill because they believe it will help them. They will lose the same amount of weight when they are given a placebo and are told that it is a diet pill; they may even experience side effects similar to those of the diet pills.

For those who have not been able to stick to a specific diet, there are now attractive alternatives. One approach is to modify the entire learned-behavior pattern that we call eating. The meal eaten must be planned ahead of time, and the dieter is encouraged to keep an accurate diary of everything consumed. This list is reviewed at each visit to the doctor, and suggestions and encouragement are offered. The dieter begins to learn his pattern of indulgence. He must elect to eat in one location in his home, and that location must be used for every meal. A single place setting is always used, and if a snack is desired, it must be served on this same place setting. Meals must be eaten at regular times each day. No other activity such as reading or watching television can be engaged in during this period. Food should be eaten slowly and chewed thoroughly. These restrictions force the dieter to concentrate on the eating situation as unique and to separate it from other daily activities. After the proper food portions are chosen, the serving dishes are placed back in the refrigerator out of easy access for a second helping.

Look for physical diversion. A tennis game, a swimming session, or a long walk will remove you from the temptation to eat. If you enjoy sweets, try to eat a fruit serving first. It may satisfy your appetite earlier in the meal. Eat slowly so that a sense of fullness can register before you finish. If lower-calorie snacks are in the front of the refrigerator, you will see them first. You can avoid tempting high-calorie foods by not purchasing any and by placing those already in the house in inconvenient places. Make your diet more enjoyable by preparing low-calorie dishes with garnishes, spices, and condiments.

If you are dining out and have no control over what is served, there are several things you can do. Trim the visible fat from your meat and remove the skin from poultry. Do not add gravy; if gravy has been served to you, eat only the meat under it. Leave some food on your plate. Assume that your daily fat allowance has been used in the food preparation and do not take any more voluntarily. Skip dessert.

Some dieters can succeed only by following a specific printed diet. For them, behavior modification is less important, and I would advise adherence to a specific printed diet such as the one included in Appendix 1. Dieters who find any of the restrictions listed above to be helpful should, of course, make full use of them, along with the specific printed diet. Guidelines on eating out are useful to all types of dieters.

It is hard to lose weight when you are suffering from emotional upset. Depression results in a reduction of physical activity. The sex drive is diminished. The lack of other gratifications associated with depression often results in more eating to "reward" oneself in a misdirected effort to feel more powerful or euphoric. Any serious emotional upset may result in a change in eating patterns.

Remember, a diet must be something you can live with, even after you have lost weight. As you approach ideal weight, you can gradually increase the portions, but if you return to your old style of eating, you will soon have your old figure again.

CHAPTER TEN

Stress and Type-A Behavior

Changes cause stress. The birth of a child, the death of a loved one, a personal injury, and changes of residence, employment, or status are all stressful situations. After recovery from a heart attack, patients often recall a cluster of stress-producing life changes immediately preceding their illness.

Stress can be defined as a physical or emotional state of tension in response to an experience to which the individual cannot make a satisfactory adjustment. It occurs when there is an uncertain outcome, the risk of harm, and no easy solution to the situation (such as flight). Everyone has felt stress at some point in his or her life; indeed, stress is a universal experience. Anyone who has had to speak before a large audience knows the sensation of the pounding heart and cold, sweaty hands caused by the stress some call stage fright. Not all stress need be unpleasant or undesirable. People seek out stress as a challenge and a source of exhilaration; witness the popularity of sky diving and horror films.

Although our days would be very bland without stress, the tension produced by it may have serious physiological consequences; that is, it may cause elevation of the blood pressure, heart rate, and blood-cholesterol level. People under stress produce more adrenaline in their bodies, which increases the demands made on the heart. Stress may also cause injury to the inner wall of the coronary artery. A rigorous debate has raged in medical circles about stress and the alterations it produces in the body, as a causative factor in atherosclerosis and aging.

What is especially interesting about life's dissatisfactions and the stress they can produce is the enormous variability of human response. One man will accept a marital conflict for many years, putting up with headaches, high blood pressure, and upset stomachs because he feels trapped. Another man may simply abandon his wife and children with little stress or remorse, only to suffer a heart attack because he cannot adjust to being denied a career promotion. What constitutes stress is determined largely by the individual's makeup and previous experience. The question is which of the multitude of life's events will be interpreted as stressful. The mark of the mature adult is the ability to continue life after recovery from stress. For some, however, dissatisfactions cannot be resolved, and so they remain like a festering sore or cancer, a continuing source of stress.

As mentioned in chapter 2, there are certain personality and behavioral traits that have been associated with an increased risk of developing heart attacks. The coronary-prone life-style is characterized by competitiveness, restlessness, and an exaggerated sense of the importance of time. People with this syndrome are so deeply involved in their work that they neglect home, family, and leisure. They find it difficult to relax and are dissatisfied with their best efforts. They eat, speak, drive, work, and think rapidly.

Working at the Mount Zion Medical Center in San Francisco, Dr. Meyer Friedman and Dr. Ray Rosenman described two personality types: type A, or the coronary-prone; and type B, whose manner and behavior are relaxed. Friedman and Rosenman classified thirty-four hundred men by means of tape-recorded interviews. Their investigations showed that type-B men with normal blood pressure and serum lipids were almost immune to coronary disease. The researchers demonstrated that the type-A individual is at an increased risk of coronary-artery disease and that this risk is independent of previously identified risk factors. Although type-A men were found to have higher blood lipids, the investigators felt that this did not explain the observed differences. The increased risk presumably due to type-A behavior is especially real in men below the age of forty-nine. Type-A behavior, incidentally, is not limited to busy executives on an expense account. A study of fifteen hundred American monks showed that type-A behavior in this group was also associated with increased coronary-artery disease.

Not all physicians are convinced that type-A behavior is a risk factor or even that it is a specific behavior pattern. Some have pointed out the difficulties in accurately classifying people. Nevertheless, the consensus of informed opinion is that both stress and personality can be measured and that they have a direct bearing on the cardiovascular system.

Equally as important as the question of whether stress causes heart disease is the question of whether you can do anything about stress. I think you can. All of us need a little quiet time every day. This need not mean a long interval; but it is important that you work into your regular daily activities a period of relaxation. Some people find that a nap or a session of transcendental meditation is best for them. But if you wait for leisure time, you may not find any.

Physical exercise is an easy way to work off stress; the type of activity is up to you. It should be long enough to be a meaningful respite—perhaps a thirty-minute period. Whether you prefer yoga or track, make sure to take some time for yourself.

There are other ways to reduce your personal stress. You cannot control every event in your life, and you are not omnipotent. Not even the most successful type A is omnipotent, so set realistic goals for yourself. Accept your accomplishments with a sense of pleasure. Reject excessive time demands on yourself. Learn to say no when you have enough to do. Many stressful events can be anticipated and avoided.

Another way to handle stress is to build some pleasurable event into every day. A hobby can mean the difference between the rat race and a sense of personal enjoyment. When you immerse yourself in a hobby, you will have a way to turn off the problems of the day. Crafts, reading, or gardening can all be tailored to fit your own schedule. Do not undertake more than you can accomplish. Relax and do only what is comfortable. If you cannot always devote much time to the hobby, do not worry. The macramé will still be there, and the garden will survive for weeks with no weeding. Just remember that a hobby is something to occupy your mind pleasurably; do not create another, more demanding full-time "job" for yourself.

I am convinced that personality and behavior play a role in the mosaic of risk factors that finally result in coronary atherosclerosis. I am also sure that you can modify your behavior so that it is less personally destructive. Perhaps the key was recognized by the ancient Greeks, who made an ideal of moderation in all things.

CHAPTER ELEVEN

Heredity and Heart Disease

Is heart disease hereditary? The answers are yes, no, and maybe. In order to understand more about this cryptic answer, it is necessary to have some background in the science of genetics. Genetics is the study of heredity and the reasons for the similarities and differences between parents and offspring. The study of genetic principles goes back more than 150 years, to when Gregor Mendel investigated the way certain traits are inherited. Mendel chose to use the sweet-pea plant for his research. Normally, sweet-pea plants self-pollinate, but Mendel used a painstaking method of artificial cross-pollination, keeping careful records of his results. After many years and thousands of pea plants, he was able to recognize the principles of genetics.

Within each living cell, each characteristic is represented by a single pair of genes, one supplied by each parent. The genes that determine human characteristics are composed of water, protein, and a chemical called deoxyribonucleic acid, or DNA. DNA is the active component of the gene and provides the basis for heredity.

Not all genes are created equal; some are dominant, others recessive. For example, if a pea-plant seed contains a gene pair that includes a gene for tallness and a gene for shortness, the result will be a tall pea plant. The tallness gene masks the shortness gene. The tallness characteristic is said to be dominant. In order to produce a short pea plant, both parents must supply shortness genes. A little closer to the reader is the characteristic of the number of fingers on the hand. If you have five fingers, you have received a five-fingered gene from each of your parents. If you had received a five-fingered gene from one parent and a seven-fingered gene from the other parent, you would have seven fingers because the seven-fingered gene is dominant. Should you then have children with a man who contributes only five-fingered genes, half of the children would receive your five-fingered gene (and have five fingers) and the other half would receive your seven-fingered gene (and have seven fingers). Were you to be unlucky enough to have inherited a seven-fingered gene from both your parents, then all of your children, no matter whom you married, would have seven fingers, because you would invariably transmit the dominant seven-fingered gene.

With this as background you can understand some of the complexities of the inheritance of heart disease and the risks of developing it. Well-defined genetic diseases that are caused by specific Mendelian traits are rare. The contribution of heredity to common diseases lies in its interaction with the environment of the individual.

Genetics undoubtedly plays a role in some cases of hyperlipidemia, or excessive blood levels of cholesterol and/or triglyceride. It is apparent that some types of excessive cholesterol are hereditary and that individuals who receive the gene for high cholesterol from both parents are more seriously affected than those who receive only a single gene. As you have learned, heredity is by no means the only factor in determining the blood level of cholesterol; most cases do not appear in family groups, and the role of dietary factors is well established. However, if it is established that the high cholesterol is caused by genetic type, the outlook is grim indeed. More than half of such individuals will experience definite heart disease by the age of sixty. Familial hypercholesterolemia, already discussed in earlier chapters, is transmitted by a dominant gene. Its frequency in the general population is 0.2–0.4 percent. However, in a large group of survivors of heart attacks it was found to have an incidence of about 5 percent.

A method of examining the genetic risk of coronary heart disease is to determine whether several family members have it. This aggregation of the disease in a family may not be the result of a single gene but rather of a combination of genetic influences affecting high blood pressure, diabetes, and increased levels of fats in the blood. When relatives of patients with heart attacks were studied, it was learned that family members were more likely to develop heart disease eventually than were totally unrelated strangers used as a control group. In studying the family history of men who had suffered a coronary at an early age, Dr. Paul Dudley White found that a high proportion of their fathers had died of coronary heart disease.

In 1966 J. Stack and K. Evans, two British researchers, studied the risks of death from coronary heart disease in the relatives of men who had had heart attacks before age fifty-five. The male relatives of these men were five times more likely than men in the population at large to develop coronary heart disease. There was no significant increase in other causes of death among the relatives studied, so we can assume we are not merely looking at a sicker family tree.

One of the best ways to examine the genetic influence in a common disease is to study groups of twins. Several countries have set up so-called twin registries. From a listing of sixteen thousand twins born between 1917 and 1927, the U.S. National Research Council examined like-sex twins who had served in the armed forces and asked them to cooperate in a study of the influence of hereditary characteristics. It was learned that there were significant genetic relationships in several factors predictive of future coronary-artery disease—for example, blood-pressure, blood-sugar, and blood-triglyceride levels. Height and weight were also interrelated.

Not all the characteristics in twins need be genetically determined. In a Swedish twin study it was learned that if one twin smoked and the other did not, lung disease was more likely to strike the smoker. In these same twins, where angina pectoris occurred, the incidence of this form of chest pain was unrelated to smoking and more likely to be genetically influenced. In chronic bronchitis, however, the reverse is true.

Not everyone has a twin, of course, so some way of predicting genetic influences in the individual would be helpful. Several clues have been discovered. One such clue, or marker, is the blood type. Everyone has a genetically determined specific blood type: A, B, AB, or O. Those with type-A blood are more likely to develop high cholesterol than those with type B or O. Other blood subgroups are currently being investigated to determine if a genetic predictor of eventual coronary atherosclerosis can be developed.

There is a genetic marker for atherosclerosis that is astonishing but nevertheless well documented. Some Japanese investigators discovered that ear wax exists in two forms: gray, brittle, and dry; and brown, sticky, and wet. They further learned that the type of wax was determined by heredity. The wet wax contains more cholesterol than the dry wax and may reflect differences in lipid metabolism. The investigators described an increased incidence of atherosclerosis in people with wet wax. This is a preliminary survey and requires careful confirmation, but it does point out the possibility of discovering clinically useful information in the most obscure situations.

Genetic studies in man are expensive and are limited by the long generation interval, so it is not surprising that scientists turn to animals to accelerate their research. It has been found that heredity may influence atherosclerosis by determining the amount of preformed cholesterol that one can absorb from one's diet. Although there may be many other factors involved in the genetics of atherosclerosis, such as dynamic changes in the blood-vessel wall caused by changes in blood pressure and emotional stress, most investigators have found it easier to measure the effect of increasing the cholesterol intake in animals. When cholesterol is fed to chickens, the amount absorbed will vary with the species of chicken. Some chickens will develop atherosclerosis; others will not.

Among rats from a given strain, the level of cholesterol is similar. Rats from one strain can be bred to react to cholesterol feeding with an increased blood-cholesterol level, whereas another rat strain will not react at all. Interestingly enough, when rats are bred with genetically determined obesity, they also develop high blood levels of cholesterol and triglyceride. The genetic determination of cholesterol level in the rat appears well established. Most rats are resistant to atherosclerosis.

Pigeons have naturally occurring atherosclerosis, and in some strains this affects all of the older birds. There are strains in which coronary atherosclerosis is rare and others in which it is frequent. No dietary or environmental factors appear to explain this marked difference, and it probably has a genetic basis. Those pigeons with a natural tendency to atherosclerosis appear to respond more dramatically when they are fed increased dietary cholesterol.

Of course, only by studying man will the problem of atherosclerosis be finally resolved. Monkeys, although they are not people, are primates, and they offer a method of studying the atherosclerotic process in ways that would be impossible in man. There is considerable individual variation in the response of both man and monkey to dietary cholesterol. On the same diet some people—and some monkeys—will develop high levels of cholesterol, and some will maintain low levels. This phenomenon in squirrel monkeys has been attributed to genetic factors. It is possible to breed groups of high- and low-cholesterol-reacting monkeys. Those monkeys that are the excessive reactors develop extensive coronary atherosclerosis after cholesterol feeding. The lesions are similar to those in humans and are potentially reversible when treated vigorously for several years with diet and drugs to lower the cholesterol level. The presence of the gene, therefore, does not mean that the situation is necessarily fixed. It is my contention that atherosclerosis in man and monkey is reversible, provided effective therapy is carried out over a long enough time period.

Is heart disease hereditary? It appears to be so in studies of family groups and in some experimental animals. Is it always hereditary? No, there are many heart-attack victims in whom no family history of such disease can be discovered. And, as we have seen, even when there is a genetic tendency to elevated blood fats and coronary heart disease, the disease itself may be reversible. A family history is a clue and a warning; it is not a death sentence, and it is not cast in stone. It must be considered like any of the other risk factors—something to discover, analyze, and react to. Although much has been learned of the genetic aspects of heart disease, much remains to be explained. In several medical centers investigations are currently under way to clarify the entire question of the genetic tendency to coronary atherosclerosis and those risk factors that seem to precede its clinical manifestations.

CHAPTER TWELVE

What a Heart Attack Is Really Like

A heart attack is an immensely personal experience. There is little in the way of preparation for this common and terrifying event that so often strikes people in the prime of their lives. As already noted, the first reaction to a heart attack may be denial: this can't be happening to me—it's gas; it's a sprained muscle; it's nerves; it's indigestion. This denial often accounts for delay in seeking medical attention. Home remedies are self-administered: antacids, aspirin, or an alcoholic drink. When medical care is finally sought, the physician may contribute to the delay by failing to recognize the seriousness of the situation or by temporizing with medication prescribed over the telephone. When severe chest pains occur, the safest response is to take the patient immediately to the nearest hospital emergency room. The personal physician should be informed, if possible, but if there is a delay in reaching him, the patient should nonetheless be sent to the emergency room and the physician contacted later.

Often a heart attack will be preceded by prodromal events—that is, precursors of the disease. The prodromal events of heart attack include a sense of severe fatigue, the occurrence of chest pains with exertion, or rapid increase in the frequency and severity of chest pains. These symptoms indicate that a heart attack is a likely possibility, and expert attention is urgently required. Not everyone with this prodrome will have a heart attack, but it does need to be carefully evaluated. I specifically exclude the telephone diagnosis from the category of careful evaluation.

The following story is fairly typical, and some elements of it apply to most heart-attack victims. Remember, when you become ill you bring to that illness all your usual personality traits, so your reactions are in part determined by the kind of person you are.

Bruce was thirty-seven years old. He was invariably prompt. His hallmark was that he always knew what time it was, and as sales manager for a medium-sized corporation, his time consciousness was a real asset. You could count on Bruce to start a 9:00 A.M. sales meeting at 9:00 A.M. sharp, even if his immediate superior was delayed. Of course, this same trait made him a terror when a report was late, because he accepted no excuses.

Unfortunately, his time consciousness did not spill over to quitting time. Some of his subordinates considered him married to the business. In fact, his wife, Celia, felt that way too. Bruce always arrived home late, usually with a briefcase full of papers that would occupy his attention for most of the evening. Bruce and Celia had three small children, and it seemed to Celia that she was always shooing the children away or admonishing them to be quiet "so Daddy can work." The result was that Celia effectively became a single parent—instructing, feeding, and disciplining the children herself.

Bruce and his family lived in a lovely home in the area most favored by junior executives on the way up. "On the way up" is the way that Bruce chose to think of himself. He had achieved a great deal since he started with the company ten years ago, but still he was vaguely dissatisfied. In an inexplicable way, he wanted more and more. Yet he could not put his finger on what it really was that he wanted more of. When he considered his achievements—and he often did—life had been fairly good to him. His job was secure; and although it was demanding, it had promise of unlimited future growth. His wife was a lovely woman, and he had no regrets that he had married her. He had always promised Celia that he would "go places." The problem, Celia often mused to herself, was that once Bruce had gotten someplace he no longer had time for her and the children. She would have settled gladly for less of his income and position and more of Bruce himself. Sometimes she told him that she missed their earlier, closer relationship, when they had had little besides each other. He would smile with a condescension that meant he did not consider the past, only the future.

Bruce found that he could often think better with a cigarette, and he had gradually increased the amount he smoked until he was a two-pack-a-day addict. He never had time to exercise, but he always had time to take his customers to restaurants. His 5-foot, 10-inch frame now carried 205 pounds rather than the 165 he had weighed at twenty-five when he had married Celia.

Bruce was always too busy to get a physical examination. But his wife was concerned and persuasive, so he finally arranged to be examined. He could not have picked a worse physician if he had tried. The doctor had been a friend in college, and the two of them spent most of the examination time reminiscing about the good old days; the examination performed was perfunctory. Still, the doctor had checked his blood pressure and intimated it was a little high at 180/95. He had also arranged for a laboratory to take some blood tests, which revealed that Bruce's blood sugar was 125 mg.% and his cholesterol was 335 mg. per 100 ml. of blood. But Bruce did not have any symptoms, and the doctor was busy, so no return visit was scheduled and no follow-up attempted after the laboratory results were returned. They were dutifully filed in the doctor's office, where they remained as essentially useless information.

Bruce went along without any further medical examinations until the day he turned forty. He had slept fitfully the night before and had decided that his most recent weight gain—now up to 230 pounds—was too much for his frame. His smoking had increased to the point where he could finish more than two cartons of cigarettes a week. He awoke at five thirty that morning and nudged his wife. He had begun to have intercourse with her when for the first time he noticed an oppressive feeling in his chest. He quickened his efforts and was aware that he was becoming really short of breath. He was so uncomfortable that he had to stop, something he had not done in fifteen years of marriage. He lay back and in a few moments felt entirely well again. He arose, showered, and dressed, telling his wife that he had to be at work early. In reality he felt so embarrassed about his failure that he did not want to face her at breakfast.

Bruce left the house and drove to his office, feeling more irritable than usual. He hated those drivers who scrupulously stuck to the speed limit, and he rejoiced every time he could pass one. He parked his car and took the elevator to the second floor; no need to walk if he could ride. Once at his desk he lit his fifth cigarette of the day.

Suddenly he was dizzy and felt that there was a tremendous weight on his chest. He could not believe what was happening. He immediately decided that there was nothing wrong; the whole thing was gas and would blow away. He called his secretary and asked for an antacid. She had worked for him for five years and always quietly did as she was asked, but today she remarked that he looked pale; she asked if he were feeling ill. Bruce became angry. "I know what I need!" he thundered. "Get me an antacid, period!" He always prided himself on his ability to make decisions, especially when dealing with subordinates. Even after he had swallowed the medication he knew he was feeling worse.

The discomfort in his chest became pain and steadily grew more intense. It began to radiate into his jaws and upper arms. Suddenly he did not want to be alone. He asked the secretary to stay with him, and he loosened his shirt and his tie. He felt very warm and sweaty, his skin was clammy, and his vision seemed less acute. The pain began to let up, and he was surprised when he looked at his watch; the whole episode had lasted about ten minutes.

What Bruce was experiencing is known as preinfarction angina, the transient chest pains that precede the development of a heart attack. Bruce did not recognize the significance of his discomfort and was angry that the pains had interfered with his usual duties. He felt better now. He admonished his secretary not to discuss the matter with anyone, and he resumed his full daily schedule.

It was during lunch that the pain recurred. He had just finished a large meal and an animated discussion with a client whose account was very important. Without warning, the chest pains struck for the third time in a seven-hour period. They were so intense that they literally took his breath away. Now there was no illusion and no secretary to send for an antacid. Bruce hated to admit to the client that he felt ill, but he knew that he was rapidly becoming so weak that he could not walk out of the restaurant unaided. He finally told the waiter that he was sick and required assistance; it was like admitting defeat.

Although Bruce had done almost everything wrong up to that point, matters improved when the waiter took command. The waiter quickly summoned an ambulance and notified the hospital telephone operator that a middle-aged man was having chest pains. An ambulance equipped for cardiac emergencies was dispatched. Bruce was quickly placed on a monitoring device that could be interpreted at the hospital emergency room several miles away. He also received oxygen to inhale through a plastic tube placed in his nostrils.

Bruce had never experienced such severe pain in his life. He felt a sensation of impending death. With his pain and anxiety, Bruce's heart rate increased. His electrocardiogram was transmitted to the hospital, and Bruce received a narcotic en route. His blood pressure was measured and an intravenous feeding device was placed into the veins of his forearm to provide access to the circulation in case this was needed. Once the narcotic began to work, Bruce felt drowsy and nauseated. He vomited several times in the ten minutes it took to move him to the emergency room.

Once there, he was simultaneously examined by the admitting intern and told he was having a heart attack; asked many seemingly senseless questions about his insurance, religion, and Social Security number by someone from the hospital financial office; and completely undressed by an orderly, who gave him an ill-fitting unisex, unisize hospital gown. This array of activities, combined with the effect of the narcotic, left Bruce quite confused.

Bruce was taken by elevator up to the coronary-care unit. He remembered thinking on the way that if anything happened in the elevator, there would be no electrical outlet in which to plug all those fancy machines. The elevator traveled four stories, but to Bruce it seemed an eternity. He was put into bed in the coronary-care unit by two nurses, one who had accompanied him from the emergency room and one, named Sue, who worked in the unit. He was struck with her youth and poise. Sue reassured him, and while she shaved his chest and placed monitor leads, she asked if she could call his wife. Her presence gave him a lift until he began to think about what she had said. "My wife, my God," he thought. He had not had a moment to think since the restaurant. He asked Sue to call Celia and to tell her that he was fine and was just being admitted for tests. This was partly an attempt to shield his wife and partly self-deception—all the more remarkable since the intern had told him fifteen minutes earlier that he was having a heart attack. Naturally, they would wait for the opinion of the cardiologist who would be seeing him shortly, the intern had said. The cardiologist on call had been notified of Bruce's admission.

The pain recurred after Sue left the room, and Bruce had no hesitation in calling her back and telling her. By now he felt really sick and was no longer trying to impress anyone. All he wanted to do was live. After the second dose of narcotic the cardiologist came in and examined him. He asked Bruce about the white lines around his iris, which he called an arcus senilis, and about the creases in both of his earlobes. Bruce could honestly say that he had never noticed either and that neither had been brought to his attention at the examination he had had three years earlier. He did remember something about the blood pressure and cholesterol being a little high, but he recalled that his doctor had not suggested any follow-up.

Shortly thereafter, his wife was ushered in to visit him. She tried to pretend that she was not worried, but the redness of her eyes was a dead giveaway. They discussed inane things, afraid to deal with what they both feared most—death or chronic disability. Mercifully, Sue came in after ten minutes and ushered out his wife. She instructed Bruce that he must rest and that his wife would be able to visit him for ten minutes every hour if they both wished.

He simply could not sleep. His mind was racing: "Why me? I've never had a sick day in my life! That checkup showed that I was fine!" Bruce soon convinced himself that the doctors were being overly cautious. Perhaps they had admitted him so as to justify a higher bill. He alternated between the euphoria of believing that it was all a mistake that would be corrected promptly and the depressing conviction that he was going to die. His work would go for naught; his wife and children would no longer have the pleasure of his company. Bruce felt betrayed by life.

The hospital routine, with its frequent interruptions for blood-pressure readings, irritated him. He resented using a bedpan. He resolved to end the whole ridiculous situation by telling the cardiologist off on his next rounds. And so he fell asleep on the evening of the first day of his heart attack.

The cardiologist made rounds at seven o'clock in the morning, while Bruce was having breakfast. "Listen," he said to the doctor, "I don't believe I've had a heart attack, and I think you should level with me. Besides, the food here isn't very good, and it's worse cold, so why are you interrupting my breakfast? I want to be discharged!"

The cardiologist smiled understandingly and said, "You really do have a major heart attack, and no amount of personal denial will change it. In many cases it takes a few days to get all the tests, but in your case the premonitory symptoms and the marked abnormalities on the electrocardiogram make the diagnosis almost certain. You can ask me any questions you like, but you won't always agree with my answers. For the time being, you are exactly where you belong."

Bruce took time to digest this answer, along with his cold breakfast. He began to feel better that day, and his eyes explored the room. He noticed that there were wall fixtures to supply oxygen and that there was a large television-type monitor on which an electron beam drew a continuous record of his electrocardiogram. When he moved in bed, the record would jump around; occasionally, if they were cleaning him or changing his bed linen, the alarm would sound, signifying that the monitor no longer registered his beat as appropriate. Bruce never completely got used to the monitor and was glad after four days when he was told he would be transfering to a regular floor.

He was pleased to be in his new room until he discovered that he would not be watched so closely and that his monitor would be discontinued in forty-eight hours. He had hated the blip of the monitor, but he had also grown to recognize that it had protected him. As Bruce began to feel better, he realized that he would survive. He began to worry about the future. Would he be able to keep up the pace as sales manager? What kind of a husband would he be? Luckily, he had the presence of mind to discuss all these matters with the cardiologist, and he received reassuring and optimistic replies to most of his questions. He was told that if he had no recurrent symptoms the chances were excellent that he could resume his normal job, and the marital relationship would not pose a problem. He did require an extensive revision of those factors that had brought him to the present situation. A long-range treatment program was set up to deal with his blood pressure, cholesterol, weight, and his sedentary life-style. The cardiologist arranged for Bruce to attend exploratory sessions with a clinical psychologist to deal with his behavior and with the stresses he would experience in the transition back to a fully active role at work and at home.

Finally Bruce realized that there was no substitute for spending time with his family; whatever luxuries he could supply them with would be less relevant if he did not supply them with himself. Bruce eventually recovered and, since his fortieth birthday, enjoys a far more satisfying life-style.

Bruce's risk category when he turned forty is especially interesting. You will recall that his blood pressure three years earlier was 180/95, his cholesterol level was 335 mg.%, his fasting blood-sugar level was 125 mg.%, and he was a smoker. If you look at the tables in Appendix 2, you will find that his risk of a heart attack was 367 in 1,000 or 36.7%. If Bruce had been treated vigorously for the risk factors that were identified at the time of his checkup three years earlier, he might not have suffered his heart attack. At the very least, he might have been able to delay the progression of his coronary atherosclerosis, and the attack might have occurred many years later.

Heart disease is not always sudden and unexpected. It often is preceded by recognizable symptoms and identifiable risk factors. If you choose to ignore these subtle clues, you may pay a price that will prove excessive.

CHAPTER THIRTEEN

Complications of a Heart Attack

After the first few critical days of a heart attack (myocardial infarction), a variety of complications may occur. One of the most common is heart failure, or failure of the heart to pump all the blood it receives because a portion of the heart wall is injured. If the right side of the heart fails, some of the blood will dam up and cause congestion in the liver. If the left side of the heart fails, blood will congest the lungs. In a severe heart attack, both sides of the heart fail.

The presence of some degree of heart failure is very common in most people experiencing a heart attack. Treatment is simple. It usually involves the use of diuretics and a drug called digitalis to strengthen the heart's contractions. The heart failure that occurs after a heart attack will be alleviated in most people if they are treated.

Another complication of heart attack, called cardiogenic shock, is more serious and in severe cases is fatal. In cardiogenic shock the heart may suffer so much damage (if, for example, 40 percent of its wall is injured) that it can no longer pump enough blood forward to nourish the entire body. The pressure falls; the skin becomes pale, clammy, and moist; the pulse becomes weak and the mind clouded; the production of urine decreases or stops. If cardiogenic shock is accompanied by severe heart failure with congestion of the liver and lungs, the outlook is poor. Should the patient survive, which is unusual, the amount of damage the heart has suffered prevents a return to a normal life-style.

Several varieties of newer drugs and artificial pumping devices are now being developed, and a more optimistic prognosis is possible for the future.

The use of coronary-care units in hospitals has improved the chances for heart-attack victims, especially those who have disturbances of heart rhythm. The value of these units has been to concentrate trained health professionals, sophisticated monitoring equipment, and electric-shock devices in one area where heart-attack victims can receive prompt and specific treatment.

A third complication of heart attack is the great variety of abnormal heart rhythms that can occur. When carefully monitored and observed, the majority of patients will show some abnormal heartbeats. But almost all harmful rhythms can be quickly and effectively treated because of their mechanical nature. One dreaded complication is the rupture of the wall of the heart, usually about four days after the heart attack. This seems to affect women more than men. It may occur if there is continued strenuous activity rather than rest and is more likely if the patient has high blood pressure. The rupture of the heart may occur in the partition between the right and left ventricles. Although rupture is rapidly fatal most of the time, the problem can be corrected by open-heart surgery if the patient survives for several months.

There is a peculiar disease called Dressler's (described by William Dressler of Brooklyn, N.Y.) syndrome, in which the pericardium—the outer lining of the heart—becomes inflamed. This inflammation is believed to be caused by an allergic reaction and is manifested by recurrent episodes of severe chest pains and fever, usually more than a week after the heart attack. Dressler's syndrome can confuse the unwary physician and terrify the patient. The diagnosis can be clarified by administering some cortisone, a drug that is often prescribed for severe allergic reactions. The fever and pain promptly disappear.

Wandering blood clots are another frequent complication following a heart attack. Clots occasionally form in the heart, especially if the muscle injury is extensive at the tip of the heart. If the clot breaks loose from the heart wall, it is pumped out and eventually lodges in an artery, which then becomes blocked. In this case the clot is called an embolus, and the organ nourished by the blocked artery suffers damage. If the artery leads to the brain, a stroke occurs; if it leads to a limb, gangrene may result. In general, the larger the heart attack, the more likely it is that a heart clot will form. Clots can also form in the veins of the legs following a heart attack. If they break loose, they float in the veins and eventually lodge in the lungs and cause an occlusion of blood flow, called a pulmonary infarction.

Still another complication is an aneurysm. A heart attack injures the heart wall, and the injured wall eventually becomes scar tissue. When the rest of the heart muscle contracts and the pressure in the left ventricle rises, this scarred portion, which is no longer muscle, bulges out like an old-fashioned balloon tire; it does not contract. The stretched-out wall is called an aneurysm. It subtracts from the heart's pumping action by its bulging and can lead to the development of heart failure. Abnormal heartbeats can occur in this area. In recent years aneurysms have been recognized more frequently by special diagnostic techniques and often can be repaired surgically (see chapter 14).

Years ago, when a patient had a fresh heart attack, he was instructed to lie quietly in bed and not to move a muscle. Unfortunately, some patients did just that, and a new disease was precipitated by inactivity —the shoulder-hand syndrome. Patients developed sore and stiff muscles and ligaments around the left shoulder, and the skin of the fingers became tense, shiny, and swollen. The syndrome is believed to be caused by abnormal reflexes and muscle spasm. In recent years cardiologists have encouraged patients to get out of bed soon after a heart attack and have permitted bedridden patients to feed and shave themselves. The incidence of the shoulder-hand syndrome has fallen remarkably and is, in fact, rare today.

There is one complication following a heart attack that can be so threatening that the patient may be unable to admit it exists. This complication is depression. In the initial phases of recovery the patient is so concerned about survival that he is unable to think of the future. As the days go by and survival seems possible, he begins to consider things more realistically. Some men become so concerned about their functions as breadwinner, father, husband, and lover that in order to stave off depression they retreat into a denial of the illness. They may demand their clothes and leave the hospital, claiming there is nothing wrong with them. They refuse to believe the evidence of their pain and their electrocardiograms.

Others are not so successful at denial and do, in fact, become severely depressed. They are convinced that their lives are over. Most patients do not fall into eithcr extreme, but, recognizing the true severity of their illness, they suffer a considerable loss of self-confidence and drive. With encouragement by family and physician, however, almost all make an adequate adjustment to the new situation.

A further complication of heart attack affects the patient indirectly. Often the spouse is suddenly made aware of the patient's mortality, which may signal a well-meant change in the marital relationship. A wife may be afraid of having sexual relations with her husband. She may prevent him from doing anything around the house, such as climbing a flight of stairs or hanging a small picture. Soon a sense of emasculation and worthlessness characterizes the recovery. This complication, which is real and frequent, can be prevented by a frank discussion between the spouse and the attending physician prior to the patient's discharge from the hospital. If the situation persists, repetitive conferences with a physician who knows both parties will prevent its becoming permanent.

The most important point to make about complications following a heart attack is that the vast majority of them are transient and reversible. Almost everyone can be fully rehabilitated and live a satisfying life with few restrictions. Despite the long list of complications discussed above, the outlook for patients who survive their heart attacks and leave the hospital is distinctly optimistic.

CHAPTER FOURTEEN

Coronary Arteriography
and Other Diagnostic Techniques

Coronary arteriography is a technique that permits the study of the anatomy of the coronary arteries in a living subject. A solution is injected into the coronary arteries and photographed using high-speed X-ray motion-picture cameras. The technique of coronary arteriography was first used in 1945 and has since been extensively improved and refined.

The most common reason for performing a coronary arteriogram on a patient is the presence of chest pain. If there is doubt in the diagnosis, coronary arteriography helps to define the reason for the pain and accurately identifies the points of arterial narrowing, should surgery on the coronary arteries be contemplated. In cases of heart disease affecting the valves or muscle of the heart the method is useful in ascertaining if coronary atherosclerosis is also present. After bypass surgery coronary arteriograms are often repeated to determine the patency of the grafts.

There are patients who do not like to complain of pain or who deliberately hide their pain from the doctor. If the electrocardiogram or an exercise test gives some indication of serious heart disease in such patients, then a coronary arteriogram may be useful. In some instances the coronary arteriogram is done because of questions raised in a partic-

113

ular type of employment. For example, if a commercial pilot develops atypical chest pains or minimal electrocardiographic abnormalities, an arteriogram may be the only way of demonstrating that he has normal coronary arteries and can continue flying.

Coronary arteriography should be carried out only in a specially equipped hospital that has back-up facilities for major cardiac surgery. The personnel must be experienced and must have worked together as a team. Obviously, one has to learn the technique somewhere initially, but this training should be at laboratories that are fully staffed by experienced arteriographers and that are designed for teaching. The nurses and technicians must be equally skilled in their particular roles.

When all these criteria are met, coronary arteriography is a safe procedure. Since it deals with patients who have heart disease, it is not innocuous; but the resulting information usually justifies the risk to the patient. In large series, about one patient in a thousand will die as a result of a coronary arteriogram. This figure is lower in the very best laboratories and higher in less experienced ones. If you ever need a coronary arteriogram, you have a right to know how experienced the laboratory is and what its mortality statistics are.

The direct method of coronary arteriography was pioneered by Dr. Mason Sones at the Cleveland Clinic in 1958. He observed that patients tolerated the dye material well and that he occasionally could thread the catheter (the long tube that is used to reach the heart) into the opening of the coronary artery with impunity. He put these observations together and had a specially designed catheter fabricated that enabled him to inject the dye directly into the coronary arteries at will. Since that time other arteriography techniques have evolved. Some physicians, like Sones, use an artery in the arm; others use the large artery that enters the leg.

There are many sources of potential error in interpreting coronary arteriograms. Unless high-quality equipment is used, the film obtained may be nearly worthless. When the technique is used correctly, vessels with a diameter as small as 0.004 inch can be seen, and narrowing can be observed in vessels that are only 0.04 inch in diameter. Even with the best equipment there are problems in grading the narrowing observed. In my own institution we use six designations to indicate degree of narrowing: normal, 50 percent, 75 percent, 90 percent, 99 percent, and total occlusion. Although these levels are arbitrary, they have great clinical usefulness. For example, vessels that are less than 50 percent narrowed do not produce symptoms such as chest pains, so it is academic if the narrowing is 20 percent or 30 percent. Yet the difference between a vessel that is 90 percent or 99 percent narrowed is very significant in terms of symptoms the patient experiences.

Another vital consideration is the number of vessels involved. If there is a significant—say, 75 percent—narrowing in a single main coronary artery, then that group of patients has about a 3 percent annual mortality. That means that 3 percent of those afflicted will die each year. An average person without heart disease might expect a 1-percent annual mortality at the same age. If two main arteries show significant narrowing, then the annual mortality jumps to about 6 percent. If all three main coronary arteries are involved, the annual mortality rises to 9 percent. Although these figures are all approximations, they demonstrate the value of coronary arteriograms in determining the prognosis and need for surgery.

No discussion of coronary arteriography would be complete without some mention of the controversies surrounding its use. There are those, like Sones, who feel that everyone with heart disease, real or suspected, should undergo coronary arteriography. Others feel that the technique should be restricted to those cases in which the decision to perform surgery has been made. The latter group considers the technique as merely supplying a road map for the surgeon. The truth, as in most controversy, probably lies somewhere in between. On the one hand, there are simply not enough well-trained teams to provide coronary arteriography safely to the 1 million Americans with heart disease; on the other hand, coronary arteriography is a useful and informative procedure providing a variety of research applications as well as information that enables cardiologists to take better care of their symptomatic patients.

One of the most familiar techniques used for the diagnosis of heart disease is listening to the heart with a stethoscope. In 1816 René

Laënnec, the inventor of the stethoscope, used a rolled-up paper tube to listen to the chest of a young girl. Physicians now use a stethoscope to determine the heart rate, its rhythm, and the quality of heart sounds. Although much useful information can be ascertained, the technique has serious limitations. Most patients with severe narrowing of the coronary arteries have hearts that sound entirely normal. Some patients do develop abnormal heart sounds, however, and a good cardiologist can discover useful clues by listening to the heart through a stethoscope. Furthermore, newer stethoscopes provide a higher fidelity of sound. The major determinant of the value of the stethoscope, however, is the sophistication of the listener rather than the complexity of the instrument.

It has always been difficult to teach new medical students about normal and abnormal heart sounds. One valuable approach is the use of a device that records the heart sounds on paper. A permanent written record is then available for teaching and for comparison, should the heart sounds change. The device, called a phonocardiogram, consists of a very sensitive amplifying mechanism that converts the vibrations of the heart sounds into a pattern etched on specially prepared paper. The phonocardiogram enables the physician to check on what he hears and to measure the intervals between different sounds. The information thus available is often superior to what the naked ear perceives. Another advantage of the phonocardiogram is that it is noninvasive; that is, the body need not be entered in order to obtain information. The sounds are recorded from the surface of the chest, at no risk to the patient, and the procedure can be repeated to observe long-range changes. The cost is modest and the technology is readily available. A phonocardiogram can be found in many hospitals and doctors' offices. Unfortunately, the amount of information that the phonocardiogram provides is based entirely on the sounds the heart produces; unless a disease changes the heart sounds, little will be learned.

The electrocardiograph, which measures the electrical activity of the heart, is a device familiar to everyone. The tracing it makes is called an electrocardiogram. Although the electrocardiograph was first developed by Willem Einthoven around 1900, we are still learning about the use of this versatile instrument. With many thousands of tracings available for study, it has become possible to set up normal standards and to decide which deviations from the usual pattern are indicative of serious disease. One method is to compare the electrocardiogram recording just before death with the anatomical findings at autopsy. The pattern of what constitutes an acute myocardial infarction (heart attack) was established in this way. It is also possible by means of an electrocardiogram to recognize the scars of a previous heart attack that healed. In addition, patterns produced by thickening of the heart walls and the presence of a thinned-out scar (aneurysm) can be recognized.

Despite these developments, it soon became obvious that the electrocardiogram can be misleading. A surprising number of people showed abnormal readings yet proved to have completely normal hearts. Their abnormality was caused by gall-bladder disease, drugs, overbreathing, anxiety, or lung disease. More distressing was the discovery that a person can have an entirely normal electrocardiogram and yet drop dead of a heart attack an hour later.

In an attempt to increase the usefulness of the technique, Dr. Arthur Masters of Mount Sinai Hospital in New York designed a simple but effective modification in the early 1940s. Before and after the patient went up and down two nine-inch steps for three minutes, Masters took an electrocardiogram. He soon learned that certain changes in the second electrocardiogram were associated with a high likelihood of coronary atherosclerosis, even if the resting record was normal. In order to increase the specificity and reliability of the test, Masters and others developed it further. A specific number of trips had to be accomplished in the three-minute exercise test, varying with the age and sex of the patient. The level of stress was about the equivalent of walking up two flights of stairs. For the individual with a critical lesion, this amount of activity was excessive. A careful follow-up study of military men showed that those with "positive" tests had a higher likelihood of developing coronary heart disease over the ensuing years than those with "negative" tests. In a positive test the electrocardiograms after exercise demonstrated changes indicative of insufficient blood flow to the heart muscle. A negative test meant that the electrocardiogram remained normal. This two-step test was still considered imperfect, however, and further experimentation proceeded.

Several research groups began to use a treadmill consisting of a moving platform that could be tilted upward in order to measure the maximum work the heart can do in young, healthy adults. The experimenters learned that the amount of oxygen used at maximal effort was an excellent measure of the degree of cardiac fitness. A natural outgrowth of this research was the use of the test on sedentary individuals and eventually on those with known heart disease. The test was soon extended to clinical cardiology practice.

The treadmill test proved more reliable than its predecessors because it provides for a high enough exercise level to reach the critical point. As the patient performs gradually more demanding exercise, the heart muscle's need for oxygen rises, and beyond a certain point, the narrowed coronary artery can no longer comply. If the patient is exercised to a much lower level of work, such as during a two-step test, then the critical level may not be reached and the electrocardiogram will remain normal.

The treadmill stress test, unlike the two-step test, is performed while the patient's electrocardiogram is being recorded. If any changes occur during exercise, they can be recognized and dealt with promptly. Normally the blood pressure, which is also being recorded, rises during the exercise. If the pressure falls, it is an ominous sign, and the test may have to be discontinued. In one group of patients who underwent a stress test and were followed for several years, those who demonstrated a drop in blood pressure during exercise had a much higher incidence of subsequent heart attack.

The safety record of the treadmill stress test is good. There is about one death in ten thousand tests and a somewhat higher incidence of nonfatal heart attacks. Considering that the test is performed on patients suspected of having heart disease, the risks are not inordinate. When the stress test is done in a setting with resuscitation equipment and trained personnel immediately at hand, the patient is doubly protected.

The natural history of any test procedure in cardiology is one of constant modification and improvement; the stress test is no exception. There are already a variety of different treadmill test procedures recommended by various physicians, differing in the speed of the treadmill, its elevation, and the duration of the testing procedure.

Who should have a treadmill test? The spectrum of opinion is broad, but some sensible generalities are available. Patients who have chest pains that mimic angina are clearly candidates and so is the forty-year-old sedentary businessman who takes up a vigorous jogging program. Some cardiologists use the treadmill to check their patients' response before and after open-heart revascularization surgery. The treadmill test can also measure the increase in fitness that occurs after an exercise training program and can identify the individual who does not improve with exercise (often the person who has a critical lesion of coronary atherosclerosis).

Patients who have recovered from heart attacks and have been referred for exercise programs often undergo treadmill tests periodically. The incidence of abnormal heart rhythms can be determined in this way, and for some, the exercise must be curtailed. The judicious use of stress testing helps the physician plan the best program for the patient.

Another extension of the use of the electrocardiogram is a small portable device that provides a continuous reading of the subject for a period of twenty-four hours. The apparatus is about the size of a cigarette case and can be worn without discomfort. The effects of effort, emotion, eating, sexual activity, and anxiety can all be recorded the moment they happen. Changes in heart rhythm and rate that occur both normally and sometimes abnormally are all documented. When the tape is played back, the events on it are correlated with the patient's diary, which specifically outlines all activities and unusual events.

This technique has produced some surprising results. When normal medical students between the ages of twenty-three and twenty-seven were studied, one-quarter had periods of no heartbeat for a 1.75-second period and about half had at least one extra heartbeat.

Another, newer, technique that extends the cardiologist's diagnostic acumen is the use of the vectorcardiogram. This instrument analyzes the same phenomenon that the electrocardiogram does—the electrical events of the heart's contraction—but it analyzes the information from a different point of view, isolating single beats for analysis. The information supplied is often not otherwise recognized, so the vectorcardiogram is in some ways superior to the electrocardiogram. The two instruments should be considered complementary to each other. Although the vectorcardiogram can diagnose certain heart attacks better than the conventional electrocardiogram, it has not achieved the broad acceptance that its early enthusiasts envisioned. Part of the reason is the high cost of the equipment as well as several competing systems of recording. Vectorcardiography shares with electrocardiography the advantage of being noninvasive and readily repeatable to document changes occurring over a period of time.

Cardiologists have also developed a new use for sound that suggests science fiction. Like radar, sonar, or the echo sounding used by the bat, which send and receive sound waves and thus determine distances, the echocardiogram sends high-frequency sound waves and receives the echoes that return. The impulses transmitted are ultrasonic, traveling through intact skin and body tissues until they meet a reflecting surface or an interface between substances with different acoustical properties. The heart structures are well suited to this type of probing, since the valves and heart-muscle walls and lining differ greatly from the blood that surrounds them.

The intensity of the echo depends on the angle of the beam, and the density and physical characteristics as well as acoustical properties of the interface. Returning echoes are presented graphically on a television screen or an oscilloscope. A photographic picture can be taken as a permanent record. By studying the patterns, an expert can determine the integrity of the heart valves and the thickness and contraction of the heart walls. The procedure is noninvasive and can be repeated at will. Research is now being conducted in the use of the echocardiogram to measure the effect of coronary atherosclerosis on the heart wall. Previously, this information could be obtained only by cardiac catheterization.

A new noninvasive technique that gives information about the heart is computerized axial tomography (CAT). This scanning device is still in development but has promise of providing some useful clues to the presence of certain heart problems. Controversy about its use for the heart is just beginning. This complex machine takes multiple X-ray slices and, with the use of an internal computer, creates a picture of the inner organs of the body. It is helpful in indicating brain tumors and certain heart defects. Unfortunately, the device is very sophisticated and expensive, and different hospitals and individual groups of radiologists have been unwilling to share facilities.

It is a truism that if a tool is available, it will be used. When a hospital has a CAT scanner, the doctors order more tests—each of which costs hundreds of dollars—and the next hospital begins to think about acquiring the device. This sort of keeping up with the Joneses becomes almost an ego trip for health professionals in some areas. Thus, the total cost of health care is raised much higher than would be necessary if hospitals and radiologists could sometimes pool technological resources.

Another recent development is the use of myocardial imaging. This involves the injection into the body of radioactive material, which becomes concentrated in the heart muscle. The heart is then photographed using special cameras. If it is normal, it acquires the radioactivity in a uniform fashion, but if the heart has suffered a previous attack, the damaged portion will distribute the radioactivity defectively. This technique can be applied while the patient is at rest or immediately after a treadmill stress test. Some types of scanning can be done on very sick patients, even during an acute heart attack, to provide evidence not otherwise available.

Several different types of radioactive chemicals can be used. Some can be given in any vein and still provide excellent myocardial imaging. Some require that a cardiac catheter be placed directly in the heart. Although neither type of myocardial imaging can be considered noninvasive, it is far more stressful to place the material into the heart than into a peripheral vein.

A further refinement of myocardial imaging involves the use of a computer. The computer subtracts first the background activity and then the effects of the radioactivity contained in the overlying ribs. The result is a clearer image of the radioactivity in the heart and a new clinically useful method of diagnosing an acute myocardial infarction in those instances where the electrocardiogram is equivocal.

CHAPTER FIFTEEN

Not All Chest Pains Mean Heart Disease

Most adults are conditioned to the seriousness of any chest pains. It is not surprising, therefore, that many minor causes of chest pains are the source of much anguish. Laypeople are not alone when they occasionally misinterpret the significance of chest pains; physicians do it frequently. You have already learned that serious heart disease can be present without symptoms and that the electrocardiogram can be normal even when all three coronary arteries are significantly narrowed. One of the most important functions of a cardiologist is to determine the presence or absence of heart disease.

It must be understood that when a typical history of angina pectoris is obtained, there is little doubt about the diagnosis. Unfortunately, many patients have very atypical histories of chest pain and discomfort, despite severe coronary heart disease. Many conditions can cause similar pains and so mimic coronary heart disease. Use of the diagnostic tests mentioned in chapter 14 will clarify the situation in most instances, but often other tests are necessary.

In a high proportion of those over the age of forty, an X ray of the stomach will demonstrate a hiatus hernia, a common anatomical finding that sometimes causes severe chest pains. These pains are often made worse by emotion or a heavy meal. The similarity to angina pectoris is further compounded by the frequent sense of relief that in both conditions follows belching. Some patients have so much discomfort with their hiatus hernia that surgery is necessary, but usually the symptoms can be controlled by diet and drugs.

Another frequent disease that can mimic the chest pains of angina is the presence of cholecystitis, or gall-bladder disease. The patient may experience pain after eating a fatty meal. To diagnose this disease properly, a gall-bladder X ray must be obtained. Unfortunately, coronary-artery narrowing and a chronically diseased gall bladder often coexist, so that the patient can have two diseases that cause chest pains.

A peculiar type of superficial chest pain is associated with an abnormality of the chest wall itself. It is termed Tietze's syndrome and can be readily separated from atypical angina pectoris because the pain can be reproduced by pressing on a tender area of the rib cage. The condition can often be resolved with mild pain medication and may be safely disregarded once the source of the chest pain has been recognized.

Some patients experience chest pains with a spasm of the lower esophagus. The spasm is a painful and powerful muscular contraction occasionally caused by the regurgitation of stomach acid into the lower esophagus. It can be relieved with antacids and changing of the body position.

Arthritis of the neck may impinge on the adjacent spinal nerves and cause pains in the arms and chest that can easily be mistaken for the pains of heart disease. The diagnosis in this case requires X rays of the spine in the area of the neck. Certain degenerative types of arthritis can affect the left shoulder and cause pains in the left arm, which may be misinterpreted.

The pericardium, or lining around the heart, can become inflamed by viral and bacterial infections and some types of allergic responses (see chapter 13 concerning Dressler's syndrome). The pain of this pericarditis can closely mimic that of coronary heart disease. Similarly, the lining of the lungs, called the pleura, can become inflamed (pleurisy) and cause chest pains.

A variety of malignant processes can affect the lungs or the structures near the heart and cause pains that are initially misdiagnosed. Once a careful examination and appropriate tests have been performed, it is unlikely that there will be any real doubt about the diagnosis.

The mind can play tricks on the unwary. A large number of patients develop chest pains because of an unresolved neurotic problem. No amount of reassurance or repeated testing will change this conviction. Unfortunately, some of these patients will have been told by their original physicians, often without objective evidence, that they had heart disease; others will be convinced that they are developing heart disease because of its presence in a parent.

One type of atypical chest pain seems to afflict young women. It is the result of a floppy or excessively stretched mitral valve. In the past, the majority of these patients were considered neurotic, but once the description of this new medical entity became known, these chest pains were recognized as part of a benign defect. The disease can be diagnosed by the presence of an additional heart sound, or click, which is heard between the two normal heart sounds.

Another type of chest pain was popularly described in World War I as "soldier's heart," because the men felt fatigued, had chest pains, and experienced extra heartbeats. The disease has many symptoms, but such a heart is not structurally abnormal. The symptoms often appear after stress and are related to emotional difficulties. The condition might be considered a "nervous heart."

Chest pains can originate in the breast. These pains are usually mild and related to the position of the body. Breast pain almost never means heart disease, but there are rare exceptions to every generality. The emotional impact of chest pains can scarcely be exaggerated. Unfortunately, even physicians develop a knee-jerk reflex response when a patient complains of chest pain. When I served as an Air Force physician years ago, I was asked to see a middle-aged woman who had chest pains. Her previous physician had referred her to me for evaluation. After I took a history, which did not suggest cardiac-type chest pains, I instructed her to disrobe and change into an examining gown. When she was ready I was surprised, shocked, and cha-grined to find the cause of her chest pain—a huge ulcerating cancer of her left breast, undoubtedly present for years!

Not all chest pains mean heart disease, but all must be thoroughly evaluated.

CHAPTER SIXTEEN

The Treatment of Coronary Heart Disease

Surprisingly, there is no direct treatment of coronary heart disease. I refer to treatment aimed at the basic disease process of atherosclerosis, which underlies the coronary heart disease epidemic. What help the patient receives is directed primarily at the complications of atherosclerosis and the symptoms they produce. The doctor treats the end result. Unfortunately, this may be too late.

As indicated earlier, the underlying disease process of atherosclerosis may be modified—an approach that until now has received inadequate attention from physicians and patients alike. Prevention lacks the glamor of cardiac surgery and is less exciting than the flashing lights and staccato sounds emanating from a busy coronary-care unit. It is dull and demanding, yet it may save your life.

If doctors do not usually treat the basic underlying cause of coronary heart disease, why are they all so busy? The answer is that they treat symptoms. An analogy would be to remove the smoke from a burning building without extinguishing the fire.

The first thing that jumps into the mind of a junior medical student when you ask him or her about the management of coronary heart disease is the treatment of pain. This reflex—assuming that the relief of chest pain is the object of the treatment of heart disease—does not stop with inexperienced students; it also extends to many cardiac surgeons and cardiologists. The pain of angina pectoris is dramatic, and the threat of sudden death is always present, so you cannot really blame the physician who considers chest pain the most important symptom to treat. Pain is what usually brings the patient to the physician in the first place, and patients are interested in its relief because they see this as the most direct way to return to a normal life. They do not realize that their old habits may have contributed to their present state, and they are, therefore, reluctant to make changes in life-style.

The pharmaceutical industry has cooperated enthusiastically with the medical profession, and the result is a wide variety of drugs to relieve pain associated with coronary heart disease. The simplest and most effective is nitroglycerin, an old drug whose use in tablet form dates from 1879. This is the same nitroglycerin as the famous explosive.

Let us imagine that a condition has been newly diagnosed as angina pectoris. We shall assume that appropriate diagnostic procedures such as a treadmill stress test, cardiac catheterization, and coronary arteriography have confirmed the diagnosis. How would the physician then proceed? The chances are that the patient would receive a prescription for nitroglycerin tablets, with instructions to place a tablet under the tongue at the first indication of chest pain. When taken in this way, the nitroglycerin tablet dissolves promptly and the patient experiences complete relief, usually in less than five minutes. In fact, if the pains are not promptly and completely relieved, the diagnosis should be reevaluated. Occasionally the first sign of an impending heart attack is the increased frequency of chest pains and the lack of prompt relief with the usual dose of nitroglycerin.

Nitroglycerin does relieve the pains, but it may also cause flushing and headache. The relationship of headaches to effectiveness is so direct that the absence of a headache may mean that the tablets are stale and no longer effective. Nitroglycerin has a limited shelf life, but newer forms of the tablets have improved durability.

Like every medication, nitroglycerin can be abused. Some patients have taken nitroglycerin as often as fifty times in a single day. Such use is rarely justified and suggests the need for other therapy. Some patients take the medication when they are short of breath; some take it after the pain has disappeared spontaneously; some swallow it whole, which destroys its effectiveness. There are also patients who fear habituation and restrict intake to periods of prolonged or severe pain. These patients suffer needlessly: their fears about becoming habituated or resistant to nitroglycerin are unfounded.

There is a time when the drug should be taken prophylactically. If a patient knows that pain is precipitated by a particular physical or emotional event, he should, if possible, take the medication before the event—for example, prior to sexual intercourse, before any demanding exercise, before testifying at a trial.

Despite its hundred years of use, nitroglycerin relieves the pain of angina pectoris by a method that is still under investigation and is the subject of controversy. We do know that the drug reduces the work load of the heart, lowers blood pressure, and dilates the coronary arteries. Nitroglycerin may also dilate other arteries and veins and cause pooling of the blood in distant parts of the body. In any case, it is effective in controlling the chest pains of angina pectoris in most of the victims who use it properly.

Nitroglycerin ointment has recently been marketed in an attempt to provide long-lasting protection from chest pains. Because the effect of an ordinary nitroglycerin pill is transient, it offers little relief, when taken at bedtime, to those patients who have angina pectoris after they fall asleep. However, if nitroglycerin ointment is applied to the skin, it is slowly absorbed, and a prolonged effect can be maintained. The ointment has been found helpful in certain cases of heart failure and even heart attacks. The drawbacks are aesthetic—the ointment is messy—and in addition, its absorption into the bloodstream is unpredictable.

There have been other attempts to provide a long-lasting substitute for nitroglycerin. A variety of chemicals has been developed under the rubric *long-acting nitrates.* Most of them are only slightly effective; few are truly long-acting. One chemical called isosorbide dinitrate (trade names Sorbitrate and Isordil) is different: it is clearly effective in a large percentage of the patients with angina pectoris. However, isosorbide dinitrate frequently causes headache and flushing. Some patients experience a sense of dizziness or weakness and may even faint. Alcohol seems to enhance these adverse effects in certain individuals. The effectiveness of isosorbide dinitrate lasts about two hours, which means that even the so-called long-acting nitrates must be administered repeatedly.

Luckily for patients with angina pectoris, the nitrates are not the only helpful treatment. A family of drugs has recently been developed that modifies the effect of the nervous system on the heart. These drugs, called beta blockers, were discussed in chapter 7. They block the nerves that stimulate the heart to beat stronger and faster. There are dozens of beta blockers, but because of excessively slow processing by the Food and Drug Administration in Washington, only one, propranolol (trade name Inderal), is sold legally in the United States. This remarkable drug lowers the blood pressure, slows the heart, and reduces its work load. It supplements the action of drugs such as isosorbide dinitrate and, in this combination, will often render the patient free of pain. When used judiciously in patients who do not have either heart failure or asthma, propranolol is safe. Unfortunately, it must be taken frequently, and it is easy for the patient to forget a dose. A newer form of beta blocker called Atenolol can be taken once a day and is currently under investigation in the United States.

Tranquilizers are often used in the treatment of angina pectoris. They are most useful when taken temporarily to help a patient over a particularly difficult period. Their casual use, however, must be condemned. All too often, the tranquilizer is prescribed by rote by the physician and taken religiously by the patient, when a little reassurance would be a more appropriate therapy. In addition, when tranquilizers or sedatives are taken continuously, there is a real danger of drug abuse, to which the patient with heart disease has no special immunity. Finally, tranquilizers have a long list of unwelcome side effects, including rashes, drowsiness, fatigue, confusion, nausea, depression, and dependency.

One of the oldest drugs in history has been used by some physicians in the treatment of their cardiac patients. I refer to alcohol, which at one time was believed to dilate the coronary arteries. The truth is that alcohol is neither beneficial nor injurious to the average cardiac patient.

Those who enjoy alcohol need not deprive themselves if it is not taken in excess. In general, a sense of martyrdom should be avoided, especially in chronic illnesses such as heart disease. Unnecessary restrictions on patients can be counterproductive. The adverse effects of excessive drinking are well enough known to be easily avoided, and most patients are able to control the dose they consume. A recent study has implied that small amounts of social drinking may reduce the risk of heart attack. The final chapter on alcohol remains to be written.

Since patients with coronary heart disease can also develop heart failure, which causes breathlessness and swelling of the ankles, their symptoms require different medications than do the pains of angina pectoris. Many patients with heart failure are treated with digitalis. In 1785 a certain Dr. Withering in England first described the use of digitalis in a patient with heart failure, which the physicians of his day called dropsy. Most of the effects of digitalis, good and bad, were described by Withering, and we have scarcely improved on his descriptions or judgment. In the following two hundred years, however, we have succeeded in changing the name of the disease and in producing dozens of different digitalis preparations. The most commonly used preparations are called digoxin and Lanoxin (trade name). The advantages of digoxin are that its level in the blood can be accurately measured, it may be given both by mouth and by injection, and it can be standardized and purified readily. These advantages are not found in other digitalis preparations.

Digoxin works by increasing the strength of contraction of the heart muscle. It also can slow down the heart rate, especially when it is abnormally rapid. Digoxin affects the peripheral veins, influences the total volume of circulating blood, and reduces the size of an enlarged heart, particularly when the patient is experiencing heart failure. All these effects tend to improve the functioning of the heart and result in a lessening of the symptoms of congestive heart failure.

Digoxin is usually administered by taking one pill every morning. Previously, physicians were taught that once the patient had been put on any digitalis type of preparation, he would require its use for the remainder of his life. This teaching has now been shown to be unduly pessimistic; it is often possible and desirable to discontinue digoxin as the patient improves. Many factors influence the amount required: age of the patient, body size, and condition of the kidneys. In general, less digoxin can be tolerated by old people, small people, and people with impaired kidney function.

Since digoxin is a drug that accumulates in the body over a period of time, it is not surprising to learn that a patient on a previously well-tolerated dose occasionally develops signs and symptoms of digoxin toxicity. The diversity of these symptoms can mislead the unwary physician. One patient may experience headache, nausea, vomiting, and poor appetite. Another may see ordinary objects with a yellow hue. The breasts in a male may gradually increase in size until there is obvious enlargement. Some patients become confused or even psychotic. Failure by the physician to diagnose digoxin toxicity can lead to serious and possibly fatal consequences.

The most serious symptoms caused by excessive digoxin are abnormal heart rhythms. Some, such as ventricular extra beats, are quite common; ventricular tachycardia or fibrillation are rare but can be fatal. The best way for patients on digoxin to avoid these problems is to have regular follow-up examinations. If there is any abrupt change in eating habits or if the patient becomes aware of irregularities in heartbeat, careful examination by a physician is vital. An electrocardiogram may provide a clue to early diagnosis, but most of the time, the diagnosis can be made by obtaining a detailed history from the patient.

Digoxin is therefore useful in many patients with serious heart disease, because it relieves symptoms and permits more physical activity. But it is not useful in reducing the progression of atherosclerosis; the basic disease continues unchecked.

If the patient's heart disease is causing congestive heart failure or is accompanied by high blood pressure, the patient will often require a diuretic—a subject discussed in chapter 7. The diuretic will help reduce leg swelling, will cause the passing off of excessive salt and water, and may improve symptoms of breathlessness. Selection of the most efficacious diuretic for a particular patient from the many available preparations requires astute judgment.

Some physicians treat their heart patients with aspirin. This is not used for pain or as a putoff ("Take two aspirins and call me next year.") but to prevent platelet aggregation. (See chapter 17.) Studies have shown that the platelets in the blood tend to come together, or aggregate, in the formation of a blood clot. Even small amounts of aspirin interfere with this platelet stickiness and therefore interfere with clot formation. Some physicians believe that as few as two aspirins a day will reduce the likelihood of a heart attack. There is a large-scale government-funded study under way to try to resolve this question of the efficacy of aspirin in preventing heart attack. But at present, this particular use of aspirin is entirely experimental and should be considered as such.

Aspirin is not an innocuous drug. It can cause ulceration of the stomach, and bowel bleeding in small, unrecognized amounts. Some patients are allergic to aspirin and suffer serious reactions. If indeed aspirin interferes with the normal clotting mechanisms of the blood, this can be a problem if the patient requires an operation.

Some patients receive other anticoagulants, such as watarin (trade name Coumarin) after they suffer a heart attack. All too often this medication is continued for months or even years after recovery. Some patients with angina pectoris are given anticoagulants as a means of avoiding a heart attack. Unfortunately, there is no solid evidence to justify either of these approaches. There are, of course, certain valid reasons for continuing a patient on long-term anticoagulation: the presence of an artificial heart valve, a clot lodged in the lungs, certain types of atherosclerosis of the arteries to the brain. The list does not include typical angina pectoris and prior heart attacks from which the patient has recovered. Long-term anticoagulant treatment for unproven indications introduces the risk of serious bleeding without assurance that the treatment will produce any improvement.

None of the drugs described above is effective against the relentless degenerative process of atherosclerosis, which causes coronary heart disease; these medications merely provide symptomatic relief. There are, however, some drugs coming into use that attempt to deal with the elevated levels of cholesterol and triglyceride in the blood. They are a step in the right direction.

When the triglycerides are elevated, a widely used drug called clofibrate (Atromid-S) is frequently helpful. It is relatively easy to take and is generally well tolerated. It produces a definite drop in the triglyceride level in most patients but has only a modest effect on elevated cholesterol levels; in a significant number of patients it has only minimal effects on both lipid levels. Clofibrate rarely restores the blood lipid levels to ideal (i.e., cholesterol below 200 mg.% and triglyceride below 100 mg.%). When used in large numbers of patients, clofibrate does not seem capable by itself of slowing down the progression of coronary atherosclerosis. In order to restore lipids to ideal levels, vigorous dietary measures must also be instituted. This has not been the case with previous studies, so failures with this medication may mean that not enough lipid-lowering treatment was applied. Only restoration of ideal lipid levels can slow progression. A little lowering does not help.

Side effects of clofibrate include a peculiar muscle ache that resembles the flu, loss of libido, impotence, and—along with most other drugs—nausea, vomiting, diarrhea, weakness, drowsiness, and rash. Clofibrate can interact with certain other drugs, especially anticoagulants, and bleeding can occur unless careful follow-up procedures are instituted. The list of possible reactions is long enough that clofibrate should not be administered irresponsibly. If the patient is on this drug, periodic rechecks of the blood levels of cholesterol and triglyceride are mandatory. If the response is inadequate, the drug should be discontinued. It should be remembered, however, that high blood lipid levels have a toxicity of their own if left untreated—and that is the relentless progression of coronary atherosclerosis. Despite the various negative aspects of clofibrate, it is probably the most widely used lipid-lowering drug available today.

Patients with elevations of cholesterol alone—who have what is termed type-II hyperlipoproteinemia—are the most susceptible to premature coronary atherosclerosis. The major drugs available to them are resins—sandlike compounds that absorb bile salts and carry them out of the body via the stool. When the lost bile salts are replaced by resynthesis, more blood cholesterol is utilized. This results in a decrease of serum cholesterol by about 20 percent. In the absence of the resin, the normal sequence is that the bile salts are reabsorbed from the bowel and fewer bile salts need to be manufactured. Less blood cholesterol is therefore necessary for bile-salt replacement.

Two resins are available for this purpose: cholystyramine (Questran) and colestipol (Colestid). The colestipol resin has just recently been released by the Food and Drug Administration and, of the two, seems to be somewhat better tolerated by many patients. Both drugs can cause constipation and gas. They have few other serious side effects, because they remain in the gastrointestinal tract and are never absorbed into the bloodstream. The biggest problems with the resins are their unpalatability and bulk. The large amounts that are necessary are supplied in powder form and cannot be fitted into a pill or capsule. They must be freshly mixed before administration. If the resins are ever to be widely used, the drug industry will have to provide improved texture and bulk.

A recently released drug for lowering cholesterol is a medication called probucol (Lorelco), on which I had the opportunity to do some of the original research. It is convenient to take, and it lowers the blood cholesterol level 15 to 20 percent in most patients. Some do not respond to probucol at all, and it does not lower the triglyceride level with any regularity. Probucol is relatively safe as medications go, but a drug rash or dizziness may occur. It is not a powerful tool for dealing with very high levels of cholesterol.

A more realistic approach for the future will involve the use of several different drugs taken in sequence to obtain the desired cholesterol and triglyceride levels. This is the method that is currently used for the treatment of high blood pressure.

CHAPTER SEVENTEEN

Anturane: New Hope from an Old Drug

An exciting new development was recently revealed in the *New England Journal of Medicine,* a prestigious medical journal with a reputation for having critical editors. The use of an old drug, Anturane, whose generic designation is sulfinpyrazone, gives promise of almost cutting in half the death rate in the first eight months after a heart attack.

In order to more fully understand the background of this new weapon in the doctor's armamentarium, let us review what happens to the almost 1 million people who experience their first heart attack each year in this country. Almost half will die before they reach any help. Some will be so mildly ill that the true nature of their illness will go unrecognized; and of those who do manage to get to a hospital, about 400,000 will survive and be discharged. The fates are not kind to all these survivors. About 47,000 will die in the first year after their heart attack, mostly because of a renewed injury to their heart—either a new heart attack or a sudden abnormal heart rhythm that kills them instantly.

The reason a second attack occurs is not really known, but researchers have been suspicious that a new clot forms and blocks a critically narrowed artery. This theory led to the investigation of methods to interfere with such recurrences.

Since 1959, Anturane had been used to lower the elevated blood uric acid levels that are associated with gout. Gout is a painful swelling of the joints that usually affects men and has as its favorite site the big toe. Somehow this location seemed humorous to nonvictims of the disease; many British artists graphically recorded the misery of such disabled sufferers by depicting an obese man with a swollen, swaddled leg propped up on a stool. The artists were amused; the patients were not.

Actually, Anturane does not relieve the acute attack of gout, but since it removes the uric acid that precipitates the disease, it reduces recurrences. As part of the research on the drug, researchers discovered that it affected the survival and turnover of platelets in gouty patients. Researchers then tested the drug in patients with cardiovascular disease who did not have gout, and the effect on the platelets was similar.

Although there has been a great deal of thoughtful investigation, the mechanism by which Anturane affects platelets is unknown, but the effects are easily measurable. Since the drug interferes with the adhesion and aggregation of the platelets, it was reasoned that it might prevent unwanted clots in the bloodstream.

Many observations are lost because they are not thoroughly investigated, but in this case further trials were performed.

In 1975 a study with the imposing name of the Anturane Reinfarction Study began in both the United States and Canada. This geographical distribution helped assure that the results would not be unduly affected by such factors as climate and local ethnic and genetic idiosyncrasies and permitted a large number of volunteers to be gathered in a relatively brief period of time.

In the study there were twenty-six academically affiliated hospitals in all; five were Canadian, the rest American. Each of the centers used the same ground rules or protocol so that the information would be comparable.

All the results were analyzed by outside medical centers of international reputation: Columbia University and Johns Hopkins University. To insure objectivity, neither the treating doctor nor the patient was informed as to whether the drug was active or a placebo.

The design of the study was rigid. Every patient took one capsule four times a day; half took Anturane and the other half took a placebo.

The patients were all between the ages of forty-five and seventy and had had a heart attack twenty-five to thirty-five days before beginning the drug. If they were taking any other drug known to interfere with platelets, such as aspirin, they were excluded from the study. The blood tests were checked by a central laboratory and the electrocardiograms were fed into a computer; thus, all these tests were uniformly analyzed.

Not every patient remembers to take his or her medicine, but the investigators were one step ahead of the lackadaisical or the uncooperative subject. They counted the unused pills that the patient was required to return at each visit. If the pill count showed that the patient was not taking at least 80 percent of the assigned medication, the patient was dropped from the study. Blood uric acid levels were also checked for evidence of Anturane's effect, in an attempt to keep everyone "honest."

About sixteen hundred patients were enrolled, and after dropouts, about seven hundred patients remained in each group—Anturane and placebo. These patients were followed for about eight months. By then it became apparent that the Anturane-treated group was faring better.

Of the hundred or so dropouts in both groups, about half were discontinued for medical reasons and the other half because of lack of compliance or failure to follow the appointment schedule. The placebo and Anturane groups were quite similar in other important respects: 85 percent of each group was male, and 54 percent of each group was older than fifty-five years. The groups also had similar past histories of smoking (65 percent) and the presence of diabetes (about 10 percent). Considering the diverse geographical and institutional sites, the similarity of the final study groups is almost ideal, which lends credence to the findings of the investigators.

The compliance of the patients receiving Anturane was excellent, measured either by pill counts or the effect on blood uric acid. The placebo group's compliance was naturally measured only by pill counts, because sugar pills would not affect the uric acid in the blood. Even new signs such as angina pectoris, which had not previously been present, were found to be present equally. The Anturane group experienced a slightly higher rate of digestive-tract disturbances, but the similarities between the treated and untreated groups were otherwise remarkable.

The treated and untreated groups differed markedly in their mortality statistics. The patients who took the placebo had a 9.5 percent annual total death rate, and the Anturane group only a 5.1 percent annual total death rate. When only the cardiac death rate was examined, it was 9.5 percent in the placebo group and 4.9 percent in the treated group.

The most striking differences were observed in the sudden cardiac death rate—that is, death within sixty minutes of symptoms. The rate was 6.3 percent for the placebo group and only 2.7 percent in the Anturane-treated group—less than half the untreated rate.

There were other, less definite trends. It appeared that placebo-treated patients were more likely to have disturbances of the heart rhythm that required hospitalization. There was a trend for the placebo-treated group to experience more heart attacks, more strokes, and more need for coronary angiograms than the drug-treated group. These differences are small and not statistically significant.

Once the observations described above became apparent, the researchers were forced to make a difficult decision to protect their patients. On the one hand, they knew that the study had lasted less than a year in most subjects, and they knew that knowledge of the long-range effects of treatment were necessary to best advise patients. On the other hand, they could not deny the apparent beneficial effects of the treatment to all of those in the study and the thousands of patients not in a study who might receive less effective treatment from their own physicians. In the end, the decision was made to provide full disclosure to all the patients and to publish the results in a medical journal. Those patients who were willing to continue with the study would have to sign a new informed-consent statement acknowledging that they understood that they might be receiving a placebo. Many patients did continue the study. The publication of the study results will permit patients who recover from heart attacks to obtain the medications through their own physicians. It was a courageous decision.

There are about nine hundred deaths a week in this country among patients who have survived recent acute myocardial infarction. Should the results of this early trial be confirmed, more than ten thousand heart-attack victims every year may be saved.

There is, of course, a natural curve to the use of every new therapy in medicine. The first reports are enthusiastic, then follows a group of confirmatory studies, some of which have less attractive results but are still positive. With the passage of time and the exposure to more patients, a pattern of somewhat more modest success almost always emerges. If the therapy is intrinsically more useful than its predecessors, it eventually reaches a plateau of utilization and value that is almost never at the lofty heights of the initial reports. Some of the new methods and treatments are gradually devalued until they disappear entirely, and then scholarly papers appear that proclaim that the author always considered the procedure worthless.

There is a time for every aspect of human experience; the studies cited above suggest that a useful technique for the reduction of sudden death after myocardial infarction may be at hand. We do not know how the drug accomplishes this, but it does have an effect on platelets, and other effects will certainly be investigated. We do know that other medications, an example of which is aspirin, also have similar effects on platelets, and perhaps future studies will show equally good or even better results with this universally available and very inexpensive drug.

What is apparent is that the pessimism and hopelessness that marked both the heart-attack patient and his dour physician years ago are no longer warranted. The outlook for the prediction and prevention of heart disease has never been brighter. Once heart attack occurs, there are powerful techniques to treat the patient and perhaps to prevent sudden death after the patient has left the hospital. In applying the incomplete knowledge at hand we can make an impact on this disease, which is a scourge of Western society.

An ancient scholar, Rabbi Tarfon, once said eighteen hundred years ago, "You are not required to complete the work, but neither are you free from making a start."

CHAPTER EIGHTEEN

Open-Heart Surgery:
Who, What, Where, When, How

Heart surgery is perhaps the most controversial procedure in modern medicine. In the early twentieth century, the heart was considered an untouchable organ by most surgeons. A few brave surgeons attempted heart operations in the 1920s, but the patient usually died. Nevertheless, the pioneers of surgery persisted, and by 1938 a successful cardiac operation on congenital heart disease was performed by Robert Gross in Boston. The results of such operations were often dramatic—gratifying to both surgeon and patient. The ailing were almost magically restored to health by the surgeon's scalpel. The operations were limited to the defects outside the heart or those easily reparable in a few moments.

Surgeons used a variety of techniques. Some permitted the doctor to interrupt the circulation for several minutes in order to operate on the heart. Another method, called hypothermia (meaning "low temperature"), required surrounding the body with ice-cold water. As the temperature fell, the brain and other vital organs experienced a gradual slowdown of activity and a proportionately reduced need for oxygenated blood. When the body was cool, a state of near hibernation set in. This technique made possible many more heart operations.

But there were limitations too; the few extra minutes of operating time that the hypothermia technique permitted were not enough for complicated heart problems. The question of time was not resolved until the early 1950s when a workable heart-lung machine was finally perfected. The machine performed the same functions that the lungs do, taking venous blood from the patient, removing carbon dioxide, adding oxygen, and pumping the blood back through the patient's body. The first models were crude by today's standard, but they did the job. American technical ingenuity, coupled with the continual demand by surgeons for more and better, soon produced increasingly sophisticated, superior machines. The heart-lung apparatus became so refined that feats of technical legerdemain became routine. Surgeons grew bolder and sought new fields to conquer.

Since coronary heart disease is so common, it is not surprising that heart surgeons began to offer patients a variety of indirect procedures. Some assumed that an inflammation of the outer wall of the heart would encourage an ingrowth of new blood vessels. They attacked the heart with scrapers, talcum powder, asbestos, and sutures, all in an attempt to set up an intense inflammation that would cause scar tissue and, perhaps, new blood-vessel growth.

Many cardiologists remained skeptical of the efficacy of such maneuvers, so a new technique was suggested: The mammary arteries run along the inner chest wall to feed the breasts in both sexes. Surgeons advocated ligating (tying off completely) each mammary artery, which would theoretically force blood to go backward; some would reach the heart. It was a safe, easy operation, since the mammary artery can be reached by a skin incision using a local anaesthetic, and the surgery would not require a direct attack on the heart. The simplicity meant that many such operations could be done by one surgeon in a morning, at little risk to the patient. It was assumed, therefore, that the patient would get relief from pain, the surgeon would be well paid, and the hospital would have a busy surgical schedule and meet its burgeoning payroll.

One group of curious souls began to wonder if this surgical procedure was all that it was said to be. Pursuing a bold plan to test the validity of internal mammary ligation, they convinced a group of patients with anginal chest pains to have the operation. Each patient was taken to the operating room and anaesthetized. A random half had their mammary artery ligation as scheduled and an otherwise equivalent group had a small cut made in the skin—nothing else. Everyone's wound was sewed up in an identical fashion. Neither patients nor cardiologists were informed as to which operation had been carried out. The patients were followed postoperatively and questioned about their chest pains. Interestingly enough, the group with the sham surgery experienced pain relief equal to that of the patients who had had mammary ligation. Needless to say, the operation is no longer available.

Dr. Arthur Vinberg in Montreal worked for many years with an imaginative experiment in dogs. He transfered the dog's mammary artery directly into the heart muscle in an area where it was needed. This technique has many limitations, however. More than six months are required for full blood-vessel connections to grow. And although the procedure has proven successful in carefully selected human patients, it is not so uniformly successful in providing a fresh blood supply to the heart as the newer vein-bypass procedures.

In 1969, Dr. René Favaloro developed an operation using the saphenous vein from the leg to connect the aorta to the diseased coronary artery below the point of obstruction. This permitted blood to bypass the coronary-atherosclerotic narrowing. The rerouting is analogous to a bypass highway that permits one to drive around rather than through a city, to avoid the congested streets. The saphenous-vein bypass is not a shortcut; it is usually longer than the natural coronary-artery route. But the flow of blood is unimpeded, and more blood becomes immediately available to the heart muscle, even before the patient leaves the operating room.

The growth of this operation has been fantastic. Only twenty-two hundred were performed in 1969; over seventy-five thousand were performed in 1977, at a total cost of $1 billion. Surgeons now do more than one bypass when it is required. One group of surgeons specializes in putting in as many grafts as necessary to completely bypass every individually narrowed branch. Their rationale is that if some are good, more are better, and complete revascularization of the heart is best. There are patients who receive as many as seven grafts.

Who specifically needs open-heart saphenous-vein bypass surgery? The main group consists of people who have severe angina that is resistant to appropriate medical therapy. There are many other less well accepted indications such as "unstable" angina. This condition exists when the patient begins to have more frequent chest pains at a specific level of activity or at a lower level of activity—for example, at rest. Aggressive cardiac surgeons have claimed that surgery will prevent a heart attack under these circumstances.

At the 1977 meeting of the American College of Cardiology, a real bombshell was dropped. The National Heart and Lung Institute branch of the Department of Health, Education, and Welfare, concerned about the mushrooming growth of heart operations, reported the results of a study it had financed. The study was designed to show the differences between medical (drug) and surgical treatment for unstable angina. Several hundred volunteers, all suffering from increasing angina pain with surgically correctable coronary-artery obstruction, were assigned to either medical or surgical treatment. The assignment was random, with equal numbers in each group; neither doctor nor patient could predetermine the treatment program. The patients were followed for three years. The results showed good news, bad news, and a surprise.

The good news was that the patients who had surgery were much more likely to be completely relieved of anginal pain. The bad news was that these same patients were much more likely to have experienced an early heart attack during or after the surgery, especially in the immediate postoperative period. Many patients, incidentally, are completely unaware of this "silent" heart attack, which occurs in about 10 percent of the surgical cases, because they are anaesthetized or receiving narcotics for postoperative pain. The evidence shows up, however, in the electrocardiograph data or in blood tests performed after the operation.

The surprise in the results of the institute's drug-surgery study was that the death rate in both groups, calculated for three years, was exactly the same. Significantly, patients with a rare type of narrowing of the main left coronary artery were excluded from this study. These patients do have a higher survival rate after surgery than after medical care, but they represent a very small proportion of the universe of patients with symptoms of coronary atherosclerosis.

It is important to realize that these results, rather disappointing for surgeons, were obtained in good hospitals with carefully followed treatment programs. There has been a disturbing tendency lately for heart surgery to spread to every nook and cranny in America, without regard to the special training of the surgeon or the appropriateness of the surgery to the patient or to the community. If there are well-trained surgeons and cardiologists and if the programs are really needed in the area, then the expansion is warranted. Unfortunately, some programs have been set up to add to the glory of local physicians and hospitals. The number of patients operated upon is small, and the deaths are distressingly high. If a hospital handles only one or two cases a week, an unacceptably high mortality rate may occur. And when a new team begins to do heart surgery in a hospital that is inexperienced in the procedure, there is a far greater risk of failure. But if the operation occurs in an institution that is accustomed to heart surgery, the surgeon is skilled and experienced, and well-trained cardiologists follow the patient's progress, then the risk can be as low as 1 to 3 percent. The percentage range is related to how sick one is to begin with. The risk will be higher, of course, with three diseased vessels and other problems such as lung, liver, or kidney disease.

If heart surgery is indicated for you, the cardiologist and surgeon should always be willing to explain why. They should discuss the risk of surgery and what there is to gain. When you decide on a matter of such importance, you will want a skilled, experienced team on your side.

One complication of open-heart surgery is chest-wall pain, which is caused by splitting the breastbone in order to enter the chest. It is often difficult to differentiate postoperative chest-wall pain from the pain of angina pectoris.

The heart may also experience a variety of changes in rhythm after open-heart surgery. Some of these are life-threatening and require vigorous emergency treatment; some are palpitations that are quite harmless but cause anxiety. Any variety of infection can follow heart surgery; the most common infections are those of the lung and urinary tract. The area of the leg where the saphenous vein was removed for the bypass may also become infected. If it does, it may take a long time to heal well.

There is another serious complication that patients are not always told about before they sign up for surgery; it is called post–cardiac-surgery psychosis. In simple terms, it means that stress has unbalanced the patient. He or she must cope with the anxiety associated with the original diagnosis of coronary heart disease and the decision to accept cardiac surgery—both severe emotional stresses. Added to that, the recovery room where the post–cardiac-surgery patient spends his first forty-eight hours is an unreal world. Day and night mingle imperceptibly; pain and discomfort are constant companions. Someone is always telling him to do something: Breathe. Don't breathe. Cough. Urinate. Swallow. There is a tube in every orifice. There are tubes in the chest where there was never an opening before. The room is unisexed, men and women sleeping dormitory-style. The patient's clothes are gone. His vital signs are measured by a nurse who is overworked and underpaid. He may see his neighbor die quietly or witness a cardiac arrest where six people pound, administer electrical shock, and stick needles into the limp, bluish body of the fellow who was just talking about his daughter in kindergarten. Resuscitation from cardiac arrest is an important way to save a life, but it is never pretty to watch, whether you are a doctor, nurse, or patient. It is worse if you are a heart-surgery patient and you realize that it could be your body they are pounding back to life, perhaps with a little less brain than you started with that morning.

All these factors combine to cause post–cardiac-surgery psychosis. The chances are that you will recover completely. You may completely forget about that period of disorientation; you may not. The following case history illustrates one manifestation of the disorder.

Albert was a forty-seven-year-old proprietor of a woman's clothing store who had always enjoyed good health. He hurt his back and was hospitalized. When an intern heard a heart murmur, I was asked to see Albert and discovered that he had a leaky heart valve and a very high cholesterol level. Albert soon developed chest pains typical of angina pectoris. A coronary arteriogram was performed, and Albert was found to have severe coronary atherosclerosis as well. Surgery was advised. Albert tolerated the operation, but for several days afterward, he could not separate fact from fiction. Now, a few years after surgery, Albert is doing well physically, but he still has a recurrent vision of a circular saw descending every night from the ceiling of his bedroom.

Open-heart surgery is a technique whose time has come. It will undoubtedly come into more widespread use. As more data is gathered it will become possible to predict which types of patients would benefit the most. There is so much emotion invested in the controversies surrounding bypass surgery that a double-blind study capable of answering all the questions about who, when, and where will never be successfully completed.

There is another aspect to bypass surgery that has received too little attention. After successful surgery, the patient may feel well and have no complaints. His coronary atherosclerosis still persists, however; and if not controlled, it will progress inexorably. Even the graft may become thickened with time. Until we resolve the riddle of atherosclerosis, the surgery can provide only a temporary respite.

CHAPTER NINETEEN

Calculating Your Own Risks

The famous Framingham study, referred to previously, collected a great deal of information on the kinds of people who develop coronary heart disease. Using data derived from this study, a series of tables were compiled that indicate the probability of developing coronary heart disease for any given person within the next eight years of his or her life. These tables are reproduced in Appendix 2. Before you begin to use them to predict your own likelihood of developing coronary heart disease, a few explanatory comments are in order.

The tables are based on data accumulated from five thousand disease-free volunteers. Seven specific characteristics for each subject were noted at the beginning of the study: age, sex, systolic blood pressure (blood pressure at its maximum), serum cholesterol level, presence or absence of cigarette smoking, presence or absence of glucose intolerance (blood sugar slightly above normal, sugar in the urine, or diabetes), and enlargement of the left ventricle (the heart's main pumping chamber), as ascertained by an electrocardiogram.

The subjects were followed for eighteen years beginning in 1948, and some developed coronary heart disease. Eventually it became possible to correlate the seven characteristics noted at the beginning of the study with the occurrence of subsequent coronary heart disease. It also became possible to use this information to predict the probability of developing coronary heart disease for anyone in the general population, provided these same characteristics are known.

To use these tables effectively, therefore, you would have to obtain some information through your physician. Failing that, various community organizations can be of help. Some YMCA and health departments offer free blood-pressure determinations, and many independent laboratories will perform the blood-sugar and cholesterol determinations for a fee, especially if you check with your own doctor first. A blood-sugar screening test may be available through local diabetes associations. If your blood-sugar level is over 120 mg.%, you should place yourself in the category "blood-sugar abnormal" for purposes of the tables.

It is important to understand precisely what is meant in the study by coronary heart disease, for that is what is being predicted in the tables. The term refers specifically to those who in the eighteen-year follow-up had a heart attack, who developed definite angina pectoris, or who died from coronary heart disease.

There are sixteen tables—eight for men and eight for women. Each of the tables refers to a specific sex and age group. By examining the appropriate table for you and finding your place on that table among the other characteristics that describe you, an accurate estimation of your risks can be obtained for an eight-year period. The tables indicate probability per 1,000. Thus, the figure 26 entered in any column means that a person with certain specific characteristics will have a likelihood of 26 out of 1,000 (or 2.6 percent) to develop coronary heart disease within eight years.

Let us look at the tables with a specific case in mind. Mr. Good Arteries is thirty-five years old. We will find him somewhere on Table 1, page 176, which describes men aged thirty-five. His electrocardiogram shows a normal left ventricle, so he places in the top portion of the table. He does not smoke, which restricts him to the top portion, the left-hand section. His blood sugar is also normal, which further restricts his placement. Mr. Good Arteries has a systolic blood pressure of only 105. His cholesterol level is 185 mg.%. Reading down from 105 (systolic blood pressure), below the blood-sugar-normal column, and across from 185 (cholesterol), the point of meeting is 6. Mr. Good Arteries has 6 chances in 1,000 (or 0.6 percent) of developing coronary heart disease within the next eight years.

His friend Mr. Artie Sclerosis is not so fortunate. Artie is also thirty-five and can also be found on Table 1. His electrocardiogram shows slight enlargement of the left ventricle (lower portion of the table), and he likes to smoke (lower portion, right-hand side). His blood sugar is a little high (abnormal), and his systolic pressure is 195; somewhat elevated, Artie's cholesterol level is 335 mg.%, which many doctors do not feel is excessive. But if we read down from the 195 systolic blood pressure (below blood sugar abnormal) and across from the 335 cholesterol, we find that Artie's chances of developing coronary artery disease in the next eight years are 312 out of 1,000 or 31.2 percent. In eight years Artie will be only forty-three and certainly will not consider himself old. But his arteries will be old. Incidentally, the average thirty-five-year-old male who participated in the Framingham study had a probability of 16 out of 1,000, or 1.6 percent, of developing coronary heart disease in eight years.

Since the tables are listed in five-year intervals, you may find that your age is intermediate between two tables. You can interpolate between the two tables and come up with an approximate figure. The same is true if your blood pressure or your cholesterol level falls between the values presented in any table. By estimating the distance between any two values you can derive a workable probability figure.

It must be realized as a limitation of the tables that only certain risk factors were taken into consideration. No information, for example, was obtained about the level of serum triglycerides or the presence of type-A personality; in fact, at the start of the study in 1948 there was little or no knowledge that these factors were important. If several of the risk factors mentioned in chapter 2 are present in an individual, then the total risk is probably even greater than that shown in the appropriate table.

Additional tables are listed for cardiovascular disease on pages 190 to 207. Cardiovascular disease encompasses the previously described evidences of coronary heart disease (heart attack, angina pectoris, and sudden death) and also includes the risks of stroke and of hardening of the arteries to the legs. This is a much broader category and if you compare the risks with those of Table 1, you will note that the risks are higher in each category. The risks of atherosclerosis are best exemplified in Table 2, whereas Table 1 is restricted to coronary heart disease.

CHAPTER TWENTY

Cooperation of the Patient

Much of this book has been concerned with the thesis that we can predict and prevent atherosclerosis. The evidence has been presented in detail. You might therefore assume that if the thesis is correct and the means are at hand to modify the risk factors, there should be a prompt reduction in risk factors and subsequently a reduction in the incidence of coronary heart disease. Unfortunately, this is not the case. We lack an essential ingredient, the cooperation of the patient—that is, the patient's readiness to do what the physician prescribes and to follow a therapeutic regimen. The old saying that you can lead a horse to water but you cannot make him drink is especially true in medical therapy.

It may be surprising to learn that less than half the patients treated for a variety of chronic illnesses actually follow medical orders. This lack of cooperation has only recently been investigated, and methods for improvement are being tested. When the doctors at a Veterans Administration hospital were asked to estimate the compliance of their own patients in following a drug regimen, they were wrong in about half the cases. They usually overestimated the cooperation of the patient.

In another case, the behavior of a group of patients with known tuberculosis of the lungs was carefully analyzed. Researchers carefully counted every pill initially distributed, and the patients were instructed to bring their pill bottles with them at each visit so that the pills could be counted. Urine was also tested for a by-product of the medication as an additional check that the pills were actually being taken and not merely discarded. It was learned that there was an error rate of almost 80 percent in taking the prescribed medication. The error rate declined after the patients were carefully taught the significance of their disease and the long-range beneficial effects of the therapy. But even when the educational program was presented repeatedly in the clinic and in patients' homes by a visiting nurse, a substantial number of errors persisted. This particular study did not include any alcoholics, drug addicts, or psychiatric patients, so the errors could not easily be explained.

Frequent errors in self-administration of medication are also found in diseases as threatening as glaucoma. The failure to control glaucoma with medication can lead to blindness, so you might expect perfect cooperation in this limited area, but you would be wrong. It is of interest, however, that once a significant reduction of a patient's vision had occurred, he or she became much less likely to make errors than a patient whose glaucoma had been diagnosed early with no loss of vision.

A much more common problem is cooperation in the treatment of high blood pressure (see chapter 7). The patient must take medication when he feels well in order to avoid future complications. It is not difficult to understand why there might be some lack of cooperation.

Since any reduction in the risk of coronary atherosclerosis requires a long-term commitment to a treatment plan, we should try to understand more about what makes people comply or fail to comply with a therapeutic program.

First of all, certain factors that are assumed to affect disease and treatment (race, religion, marital status, socioeconomic group, geographic location, mode of living) have little bearing on long-range cooperation.

If the patient's disease causes no symptoms, then he is less likely to follow the treatment plan correctly (as noted in the case of high blood pressure), and he is more likely to drop out of treatment entirely. This is true even if a special attempt is made to bring the medication to the patient at his place of employment. In a study in Canada, steelworkers who had high blood pressure were offered treatment either by their family doctor or at work. The belief was that the increased convenience and the reduction in time required would result in far better coopera- tion. When the study was completed, it was apparent that offering the treatment to the men at work did not result in a significantly greater degree of cooperation.

A patient is less likely to follow a treatment regimen if the medica- tion interrupts his life-style. He is also less likely to persist if neither he nor his physician really believes in the efficacy of the approach. The best example of the latter is cigarette smoking. If the physician smokes, the patient will find it much harder to stop. Furthermore, if immediate family members are unsympathetic to the treatment, then the treat- ment is more likely to be discontinued. This is particularly true for special diets, exercise programs, and drugs taken at mealtimes.

Some noncompliance factors are specific to drug therapy. One of these is cost. The more expensive the medicine, the less the long-range cooperation. Another factor is a complicated drug regimen requiring several medications given at different times. As the sequence becomes more complicated, it is more likely to fail. Also, if the drug tastes bad or if the patient experiences side effects, the therapeutic schedule will not be followed; this point has particular relevance in the treatment of high blood-cholesterol levels.

Other factors also affect cooperation. For example, the desire to stop smoking is effectively counterbalanced by a well-financed industry that manufactures, markets, and advertises cigarettes. There are social mores about eating that interfere with a low-calorie, low-cholesterol, low-saturated-fat diet. Despite all the talk about the desirability of being thin and the multibillion-dollar diet fad, Americans every year eat about sixty pounds of fat—that is, fat products per se, not the fat normally present in meat, cheese, milk, and the like. A major factor in this fat consumption is the rapid growth of processed foods manufac- tured with fats.

There are ways out of this morass. Investigating lack of patient cooperation, a neighborhood health center discovered that more than one-third of the appointments were broken, and it therefore began contacting patients before their scheduled visits; this resulted in far fewer absences. Certainly critical to any improvement in cooperation is better physician-patient communication. The patient often does not know what the physician is saying, and often the physician says too little. When other health professionals—nurses, dietitians, paramedical personnel—are utilized to help educate the patient, cooperation is increased and fewer errors result. The patient should be told exactly what the various pills and dietary measures are designed to accomplish. A good trick is to have him repeat the information before leaving the doctor's office. Unfortunately, many physicians faced with an uncooperative patient simply refuse to treat him further. Their approach suggests that the problem is unique to the patient; in reality, it is shared.

If the patient is going to be successful at long range reduction of risks, he needs a game plan. The drugs must be conveniently clued into meals and normal sleep patterns so that there is less disruption of daily routine. The strong support of family members must be encouraged. If you are in a high-risk group, you should be treated by a doctor interested in preventive medicine. Be sure to ask whatever questions arise in your mind; unless you clearly understand the purpose of the drugs, you will soon be making errors. Decide what you can and cannot do. If there is something that you are unable to accept, discuss it with your physician so that the two of you can reach a compromise. It is much easier to cooperate in a short-term illness; but risk reduction means a lifetime commitment.

Society too has a role in helping patient cooperation. There is a role for the pharmaceutical industry in improving the design of tablets so that they can be readily identified, thus removing one source of patient error. A good deal of preliminary work has already been done along these lines. There is also a role for physicians, who should become more oriented to the values of preventive medicine and using other health personnel and who should improve their patients' concepts of their diseases and required treatment. There is a role too for the mass media, which should distribute information on preventive medicine in an understandable way and help motivate those who are ready for a specific behavioral modification. There is a role for consumer groups more attuned to the need for preventive changes in risk factors to form organizations dealing with such matters as exercise classes or a redefinition of the amount of fats in margarine, hot dogs, and prime meats.

In the future we will probably have more organized programs, which are now in the process of development and will be largely government financed. If you choose to wait, the future programs may come too late to do you much good. Only if you take the responsibility for your own health can the appropriate actions be taken now.

APPENDICES

A Cereal-Based Diet

The purpose of this diet* is twofold: (1) to lower body weight through reduced caloric intake, and (2) to lower the blood-cholesterol level through reduced intake of saturated fats and cholesterol. Being overweight and having high blood-cholesterol levels are considered major risk factors in the development of atherosclerosis.

The cereal-based diet is organized around six major groups of permissible foods: breads and cereals; vegetables; milk and milk products; meat, fish, and meat substitutes; fruits and fruit juices; and fats and oils. Each meal has specific group requirements, indicated below in the Basic Meal Plan. The six food groups, which follow, contain lists of foods with precise amounts noted for each serving. Although each food group is large enough to permit great variety in menu planning, a number of cross-group substitutions are possible, supplemented by a Free Foods list. Acceptable substitutions are listed under the individual food groups.

The following instructions will help you to carry out the program systematically:

1. Follow your meal pattern exactly. Do not carry foods over from one meal to the next. Eat all the foods allowed at each meal.
2. Weigh or measure foods when eating at home.
3. Eat at regular times each day.
4. Record daily all foods eaten and the quantity consumed.
5. Eat slowly and chew food thoroughly.
6. Try to avoid a menu that is different from that of the rest of the family.

*The diet is discussed more fully in *Dr. Nash's Natural Diet Book,* Grosset and Dunlap, 1978.

159

BASIC MEAL PLAN

	FOOD GROUP	AMOUNT PERMITTED
Breakfast	fruits and fruit juices	1 serving*
	breads and cereals	2 servings
	milk and milk products	½ cup skim milk or** equivalent
Lunch	meat, fish, and meat substitutes	2 oz.
	breads and cereals	2 servings
	vegetables, "A" list	as desired
	fats and oils	1 serving
	fruits and fruit juices	1 serving
	milk and milk products	½ cup skim milk or equivalent
Dinner	meat, fish, and meat substitutes	3 oz.
	breads and cereals	2 servings
	vegetables, "A" list	as desired
	fats and oils	1 serving
	fruits and fruit juices	1 serving
	milk and milk products	½ cup skim milk or equivalent
Snack	breads and cereals***	1 serving
	milk and milk products	½ cup skim milk or equivalent

*A serving is defined within the individual food groups.

**A total of 2 cups of skim milk or its equivalent is allowed daily, distributed as the dieter wishes.

***A single drink can be substituted for the cereal serving of the snack. A one-ounce portion of bourbon or brandy is equivalent in calories to the cereal serving.

FOOD GROUPS

BREADS AND CEREALS

There are four subcategories of this group. Substitutions may be introduced from the "B" Vegetables list. Seven bread servings per day are permitted.

BREADS	AMOUNT EQUAL TO 1 BREAD SERVING
bagel	½
biscuit (2-in. diam.)	1*
bread: enriched white, rye, wheat, pumpernickel, Italian, French, raisin	1 slice
bread crumbs: dry, grated	3 tbs.
bread stick: large	1
cornmeal	3 tbs.
crackers:	
graham (2½ in. sq.)	2
matzo (6 in. × 6 in.)	1
melba toast	4
oyster	½ cup
Ritz	2
round, thin	6
Rye-Krisp	3
rye thin	10
saltine	5
soda	3
wheat thin	12
English muffin	½
flour	3 tbs.
grits: cooked	½ cup
macaroni: cooked	½ cup
muffin (3-in. diam.)	1*
noodles: cooked	½ cup
pancake (4-in. diam.)	2*
rice	½ cup

BREADS	AMOUNT EQUAL TO 1 BREAD SERVING
roll:	
hamburger	½
hard, large	½
hard, small	1
hot dog	½
spaghetti: cooked	½ cup
waffle (6-in. diam.)	½ *

CEREALS	AMOUNT EQUAL TO 1 BREAD SERVING

Dry

All Bran	½ cup
Bran Flakes	¾ cup
Cheerios	1 cup
Cornflakes	¾ cup
Grape Nut Flakes	½ cup
Grape Nuts	¼ cup
Life	1 cup
natural cereals (without nuts)	⅓ cup
Post Toasties	1 cup
puffed rice	½ cup
puffed wheat	½ cup
Raisin Bran	½ cup
Rice Krispies	¾ cup
shredded wheat	1 biscuit
Special K	1 cup
spoon-size shredded wheat	½ cup
Wheat Chex	⅓ cup
Wheaties	¾ cup

Cooked

all cooked cereals	½ cup

*The amount given is equal to 1 bread serving plus 1 fat serving.

HIGH-CARBOHYDRATE VEGETABLES	AMOUNT EQUAL TO 1 BREAD SERVING

Starchy vegetables can be considered cereal equivalents for the purposes of this diet. It is a simplistic but pragmatic compromise.

beans:	
baked (no pork or molasses)	¼ cup
dried, cooked	½ cup
lima	½ cup
corn:	
small (4-in. ear)	1
whole kernel	⅓ cup
mixed	⅔ cup
parsnips	⅔ cup
peas: dried, cooked	½ cup
potatoes:	
mashed	½ cup
sweet	¼ cup
white (2-in. diam.)	1

"B" VEGETABLES

"B" vegetables contain some carbohydrate. They should be eaten in ½-cup servings and should be substituted for ½ of a bread serving. Starchy vegetables were listed above.

beets	½ cup
carrots	½ cup
onions	½ cup
pumpkin	½ cup
rutabaga	½ cup
squash, winter	½ cup
turnips	½ cup

MISCELLANEOUS CEREAL EQUIVALENTS	AMOUNT EQUAL TO 1 BREAD SERVING
animal crackers	7
cake: angel food	1½- in. slice
fig bar	1
gelatin	½ cup
ginger snaps	4 small
popcorn, plain	1 cup
pretzels:	
Dutch	1
three-ring	6
pudding, low-calorie instant with skim milk	1 cup
soup, commercial, prepared with water; vegetable, vegetarian vegetable	1 cup

VEGETABLES

Vegetables may be seasoned freely with lemon juice, chopped chives, green pepper, and various spices to enhance their flavor. They may be combined with bouillon to make a variety of soups. If fat or oil is used in preparation, the amount used must be deducted from the fat allowance for that meal.

The "A" vegetables are low in calories and contain negligible amounts of carbohydrate, protein, or fat. Therefore, they may be eaten freely; that is, in normal amounts at mealtime or between meals if desired.

"A" VEGETABLES

artichokes
asparagus
bean sprouts
beet greens
broccoli
brussels sprouts
cabbage
cauliflower
celery
chicory

Chinese cabbage
collard greens
cucumbers
dandelion greens
eggplant
endive
escarole
kale
lettuce
mushrooms

mustard greens
okra
pepper, green
pickle, sour
radishes
romaine
sauerkraut
scallions
spinach

squash, summer, yellow
   crookneck, straightneck
   zucchini
Swiss chard
string beans, green, yellow
tomatoes
turnip greens
watercress

MILK AND MILK PRODUCTS

Items in this food group may be served as is or used in food preparation; in the latter case, the amount used must be deducted from the daily allowance, which is 2 cups of skim milk or its equivalent. This amount may be distributed among the meals as desired.

MILK AND MILK PRODUCTS	AMOUNT EQUAL TO 1 SKIM MILK SERVING (1 CUP)
buttermilk (from skim milk)	1 cup
cottage cheese:	
creamed	½ cup*
dry curd	⅓ cup
uncreamed	⅓ cup
ice milk	½ cup*
milk:	
99% fat-free	1 cup
skim, liquid	1 cup
skim, dry, powdered	⅓ cup dry
skim, evaporated	½ cup undiluted
2% fat	1 cup*
sherbet	⅓ cup
yogurt, unflavored (from skim milk)	1 cup*

MEAT, FISH, AND MEAT SUBSTITUTES

Select lean, well-trimmed cuts of meat when fresh or frozen. Visible fat should be removed before preparation. Meat may be baked, broiled, boiled, or roasted. It should not bake or roast in its own juices; a rack should be used. Brown meats under the broiler. Additional fat used for browning must be within the fat allowance.

Fish should preferably be fresh or canned. When canned in oil, it must be well drained.

Items in the "A" list are significantly lower in fat and cholesterol than those in the "B" list. Most of your selections should be made from the "A" list, with the "B" list used occasionally for variety. The "C" list may be used freely.

For this food group, the daily allowance (after cooking) is 5 ounces: 2 at lunch, 3 at dinner. Allow for shrinkage and waste. For each cooked 3-ounce portion, buy 5 ounces of raw meat with bone or 4 ounces boneless.

Typical 3-ounce cooked servings:

½ breast of 3-pound chicken
    leg and thigh of 3-pound chicken
¾ cup chicken meat, loosely packed
2 slices roast beef (4 in. × 2 in. × ¼ in.)
¾ cup canned tuna
¾ cup canned salmon

"A" LIST

Beef
arm
round-bone sirloin
tenderloin

Fish
all fish; limit shellfish to once a week

Poultry
chicken (meat only; avoid skin)
turkey (meat only; avoid skin)

Veal
all cuts

"B" LIST

Beef

chipped beef, dried
chuck rib
club
corned beef, canned, *lean*
flank
porterhouse
round, lean
rump
short plate
sirloin

Lamb

leg
loin

Pork

Boston butt
ham, *lean*
loin

"C" LIST

(substitutes for meat, fish, or fowl)

	AMOUNT EQUAL TO 1 2-OZ. MEAT SERVING
beans: dried, cooked	1 cup
cottage cheese, creamed	½ cup
low-fat cheese (less than 5% fat; see label)	2 oz.
mozzarella cheese	1½ oz.
peas: dried, cooked	1 cup
yogurt, unflavored (from skim milk)	1 cup

FRUITS AND FRUIT JUICES

Use fresh, dried, cooked, canned, or frozen fruit or juice to which neither sugar nor syrup has been added; the item should be labeled "unsweetened." If fruits have been canned in syrup, rinse them thoroughly with water before serving. Do not add sugar or honey to fresh fruit. The daily allowance for this group is 3 servings, of which at least 1 serving should be a citrus fruit or juice.

FRUITS	AMOUNT EQUAL TO 1 SERVING*
apple, small	1
applesauce	⅓ cup
apricots: fresh, canned, or dried	4 halves
banana, small	½
blackberries	1 cup
blueberries	½ cup
cantaloupe	¼
cherries	12
dates	2
figs:	
canned (medium size)	3
dried (small)	1
fruit cocktail	½ cup
grapefruit:	
whole, small	½
sections	½ cup
grapes:	
large	12
small	20
honeydew	⅛
nectarine, medium	1
orange, fresh, medium	1
peach, medium	1
pear	2 halves
pineapple:	
rings	2
chunks	⅓ cup
plums, medium	2
prunes, dried	2
raisins	2 tbs.
raspberries	¾ cup
strawberries	1 cup
watermelon, diced	1 cup

*Unless otherwise indicated, amounts for fresh portions and canned portions are the same.

FRUIT JUICES	AMOUNT EQUAL TO 1 FAT SERVING
apple	⅓ cup
cider	⅓ cup
cranberry	½ cup
grape	¼ cup
grapefruit	½ cup
orange	½ cup
pineapple	⅓ cup
prune	¼ cup

FATS AND OILS

Several items listed below—avocado and nuts, for example—are not usually thought of as fats or oils. However, these foods are so rich in fats and oils that, for purposes of the diet, it is useful to classify them in this category. Two fat servings per day are permitted.

FATS AND OILS	AMOUNT EQUAL TO 1 FAT SERVING
avocado (4 in. long)	⅛
margarine*	1 tsp.
mayonnaise	2 tsp.
nuts (no coconut)	1 tbs.
olives, small	5
peanut butter	2 tsp.
salad dressing, commercial (no sour cream)	1 tbs.
vegetable oils: corn, cottonseed, safflower, sunflower, and soybean only	1 tsp.

*Margarine must be made from one of the five listed vegetable oils. The first ingredient mentioned on the label (i.e., the predominant ingredient) must be liquid oil—not hardened, partially hardened, or hydrogenated.

FREE FOODS

Use as desired.

artificial sweeteners
bouillon
carbonated beverages, sugarless
coffee
chewing gum, sugarless
gelatin, unsweetened
horseradish
lemon juice

mustard
soy sauce
spices, herbs, and flavorings
tea
vegetables in "A" list
vegetable juice
vinegar

FOODS TO AVOID

bacon
butter
cheese made from cream or whole
    milk
chocolate
cream: sour, sweet
creamed dishes and soups
cream substitutes
egg yolk (check ingredients of
    commercial mixes)
fat, visible on meat
fish: caviar, mackerel, roe, sardines

frozen and packaged dinners
ice cream
meat: canned, cold cuts, commercially
    fried, fatty, frozen in gravy or sauce,
    hot dogs, lunch meat, organs, spare
    ribs
milk: condensed, dried, evaporated,
whole, whole-milk drinks
sausage
sauces, unless made with allowed
    fat and skimmed stock
poultry: duck, goose, skin
whipped toppings, commercial

SUGGESTIONS FOR RESTAURANT DINING

First course: clear soup, fruit cup, tomato juice, vegetable juice cocktail,
    relish plate
Salads: tossed salads with allowed dressing served separately
Entrees: fish or chicken (not fried); sliced turkey, veal, or roast beef; lean
    corned beef; fruit, gelatin, fish, or seafood salad (dressing served sepa-
    rately); vegetable plate (no butter). If dieter's plate is available, it should
    not exceed 360 calories (check to be sure that it does not include foods
    that are not allowed on your diet, such as eggs).

Desserts: A serving of fruit or 1 bread serving may be used for sherbet, gelatin, or unfrosted angel-food cake.

CHOLESTEROL TABLE

	AMOUNT OF CHOLESTEROL IN 100 GRAMS, EDIBLE PORTION, IN MILLIGRAMS
Beef, raw:	
with bone	70
without bone	70
Brains, raw	greater than 2,000
Butter	250
Caviar or fish roe	greater than 300
Cheese:	
cheddar	100
cottage, creamed	15
cream	120
other (25%–30% fat)	85
Cheese spread	65
Chicken, flesh only, raw	60
Crab:	
in shell	125
meat only	125
Egg, whole	550
Egg white	0
Egg yolk:	
fresh	1,500
frozen	1,280
dried	2,950
Fish:	
steak	70
fillet	70
Heart, raw	150
Ice cream	45
Kidney, raw	375

	AMOUNT OF CHOLESTEROL IN 100 GRAMS, EDIBLE PORTION, IN MILLIGRAMS
Lamb, raw:	
with bone	70
without bone	70
Lard and other animal fat	95
Liver, raw	300
Lobster:	
whole	200
meat only	200
Margarine:	
all vegetable fat	0
two-thirds animal fat, one-third vegetable fat	65
Milk:	
fluid, whole	11
dried, whole	85
fluid, skim	3
Oysters:	
in shell	greater than 200
meat only	greater than 200
Pork:	
with bone	70
without bone	70
Shrimp:	
in shell	125
flesh only	125
Sweetbreads (thymus)	250
Veal:	
with bone	90
without bone	90

DESIRABLE WEIGHTS FOR MEN AND WOMEN

According to Height and Frame. Ages 25 and Over

HEIGHT IN SHOES	WEIGHT IN POUNDS (IN INDOOR CLOTHING)		
	SMALL FRAME	MEDIUM FRAME	LARGE FRAME
	MEN		
5 ' 2"	112–120	118–129	126–141
3"	115–123	121–133	129–144
4"	118–126	124–136	132–148
5"	121–129	127–139	135–152
6"	124–133	130–143	138–156
7"	128–137	134–147	142–161
8"	132–141	138–152	147–166
9"	136–145	142–156	151–170
10"	140–150	146–160	155–174
11"	144–154	150–165	159–179
6' 0"	148 158	154–170	164–184
1"	152–162	158–175	168–189
2"	156–167	162–180	173–194
3"	160–171	167–185	178–199
4"	164–175	172–190	182–204
	WOMEN		
4' 10"	92–98	96–107	104–119
11"	94–101	98–110	106–122
5' 0"	96–104	101–113	109–125
1"	99–107	104–116	112–128
2"	102–110	107–119	115–131
3"	105–113	110–122	118–134
4"	108–116	113–126	121–138
5"	111–119	116–130	125–142
6"	114–123	120–135	129–146
7"	118–127	124–139	133–150
8"	122–131	128–143	137–154
9"	126–135	132–147	141–158
10"	130–140	136–151	145–163
11"	134–144	140–155	149–168
6' 0"	138–148	144–159	153–173

TABLE 1.

Coronary Heart Disease

ABBREVIATIONS FOR TABLES

Chol: Cholesterol

SBP: Systolic blood pressure

LVH: Left ventricular hypertrophy
       (an enlargement of the left ventricle)

ECG: Electrocardiogram

TABLE 1A. PROBABILITY (PER 1,000) OF DEVELOPING CORONARY

DOES NOT SMOKE CIGARETTES

NO ENLARGED HEART BY ECG

	SBP	105	120	135	150	165	180	195
	Chol.							
GLUCOSE	185	6	7	8	10	11	14	16
INTOLERANCE	210	8	10	11	14	16	19	23
ABSENT	235	11	14	16	19	23	27	32
	260	16	19	23	27	32	38	45
	285	23	27	32	38	45	54	64
	310	32	38	45	54	64	75	88
	335	45	54	64	75	88	103	121

	SBP	105	120	135	150	165	180	195
	Chol.							
GLUCOSE	185	7	8	10	12	14	17	20
INTOLERANCE	210	10	12	14	17	20	24	29
PRESENT	235	14	17	20	24	29	34	40
	260	20	24	29	34	40	48	57
	285	29	34	40	48	57	67	79
	310	40	48	57	67	79	93	109
	335	57	67	79	93	109	127	148

ECG SHOWS ENLARGED HEART (LVH)

	SBP	105	120	135	150	165	180	195
	Chol.							
GLUCOSE	185	10	11	13	16	19	23	27
INTOLERANCE	210	13	16	19	23	27	32	38
ABSENT	235	19	23	27	32	38	45	53
	260	27	32	38	45	53	63	74
	285	38	45	53	63	74	87	103
	310	53	63	74	87	103	120	140
	335	74	87	103	120	140	163	188

	SBP	105	120	135	150	165	180	195
	Chol.							
GLUCOSE	185	12	14	17	20	24	28	34
INTOLERANCE	210	17	20	24	28	34	40	47
PRESENT	235	24	28	34	40	47	56	66
	260	34	40	47	56	66	78	92
	285	47	56	66	78	92	108	126
	310	66	78	92	108	126	147	170
	335	92	108	126	147	170	197	226

*Framingham men aged 35 years have an average SBP of 127 mm. Hg and an average serum cholesterol of 220 mg.%; 70% smoke cigarettes, 0.0% have definite LVH by ECG, and 1.7%

SMOKES CIGARETTES

NO ENLARGED HEART BY ECG

SBP	105	120	135	150	165	180	195
Chol.							
185	9	10	12	15	18	21	25
210	12	15	18	21	25	30	35
235	18	21	25	30	35	42	49
260	25	30	35	42	49	58	69
285	35	42	49	58	69	81	95
310	49	58	69	81	95	112	130
335	69	81	95	112	130	152	176

SBP	105	120	135	150	165	180	195
Chol.							
185	11	13	16	19	22	26	31
210	16	19	22	26	31	37	44
235	22	26	31	37	44	52	61
260	31	37	44	52	61	72	85
285	44	52	61	72	85	100	117
310	61	72	85	100	117	137	159
335	85	100	117	137	159	184	212

ECG SHOWS ENLARGED HEART (LVH)

SBP	105	120	135	150	165	180	195
Chol.							
185	15	17	21	25	29	35	41
210	21	25	29	35	41	49	58
235	29	35	41	49	58	68	80
260	41	49	58	68	80	94	111
285	58	68	80	94	111	129	151
310	80	94	111	129	151	175	202
335	111	129	151	175	202	232	265

SBP	105	120	135	150	165	180	195
Chol.							
185	18	22	26	31	37	43	51
210	26	31	37	43	51	61	72
235	37	43	51	61	72	84	99
260	51	61	72	84	99	116	136
285	72	84	99	116	136	158	183
310	99	116	136	158	183	211	242
335	136	158	183	211	242	275	312

have glucose intolerance. At these average values the probability of developing coronary heart disease in eight years is 16/1000.

TABLE 1B. PROBABILITY (PER 1,000) OF DEVELOPING CORONARY

DOES NOT SMOKE CIGARETTES

NO ENLARGED HEART BY ECG

	SBP	105	120	135	150	165	180	195
	Chol.							
GLUCOSE	185	11	14	16	19	23	27	32
INTOLERANCE	210	15	18	22	26	31	37	43
ABSENT	235	21	25	29	35	41	49	58
	260	28	33	40	47	55	65	77
	285	38	45	53	63	74	87	102
	310	51	60	71	83	98	115	134
	335	68	80	94	110	129	150	174

	SBP	105	120	135	150	165	180	195
	Chol.							
GLUCOSE	185	14	17	20	24	29	34	40
INTOLERANCE	210	19	23	27	32	38	46	54
PRESENT	235	26	31	37	44	52	61	72
	260	35	42	49	58	69	81	95
	285	47	56	66	78	91	107	125
	310	63	74	88	103	120	140	163
	335	84	99	116	135	157	182	210

ECG SHOWS ENLARGED HEART (LVH)

	SBP	105	120	135	150	165	180	195
	Chol.							
GLUCOSE	185	19	23	27	32	38	45	53
INTOLERANCE	210	26	30	36	43	51	60	71
ABSENT	235	35	41	49	57	68	80	94
	260	46	55	65	77	90	106	124
	285	62	73	86	101	119	138	161
	310	83	97	114	133	155	179	207
	335	109	128	149	173	199	229	262

	SBP	105	120	135	150	165	180	195
	Chol.							
GLUCOSE	185	24	28	34	40	47	56	66
INTOLERANCE	210	32	38	45	53	63	74	88
PRESENT	235	43	51	60	71	84	99	116
	260	58	68	80	95	111	130	151
	285	77	91	106	124	145	168	195
	310	102	119	139	162	187	216	247
	335	134	156	180	208	239	272	309

*Framingham men aged 40 years have an average SBP of 129 mm. Hg and an average serum cholesterol of 228 mg.%; 70% smoke cigarettes, 0.3% have definite LVH by ECG, and 3.3%

SMOKES CIGARETTES

NO ENLARGED HEART BY ECG

SBP	105	120	135	150	165	180	195
Chol.							
185	18	21	25	29	35	41	49
210	24	28	33	40	47	56	66
235	32	38	45	53	63	74	87
260	43	51	60	71	83	98	115
285	57	68	80	94	110	129	150
310	77	90	106	124	144	167	194
335	101	119	138	161	186	215	246

SBP	105	120	135	150	165	180	195
Chol.							
185	22	26	31	37	44	52	61
210	30	35	42	49	58	69	81
235	40	47	56	66	78	91	107
260	53	63	75	88	103	120	141
285	71	84	99	116	135	157	182
310	95	111	130	151	175	202	232
335	124	145	168	195	224	256	291

ECG SHOWS ENLARGED HEART (LVH)

SBP	105	120	135	150	165	180	195
Chol.							
185	29	35	41	49	58	68	80
210	39	47	55	65	77	90	106
235	53	62	73	86	101	119	139
260	70	83	97	114	133	155	179
285	93	109	128	149	173	199	229
310	123	143	166	192	221	253	288
335	160	185	213	244	278	315	355

SBP	105	120	135	150	165	180	195
Chol.							
185	36	43	51	61	71	84	99
210	49	58	68	81	95	111	130
235	65	77	91	106	124	145	168
260	87	102	120	139	162	188	216
285	115	134	156	181	208	239	273
310	150	174	201	231	263	299	338
335	193	222	254	290	327	367	409

have glucose intolerance. At these average values the probability of developing coronary heart disease in eight years is 34/1000.

TABLE 1C. PROBABILITY (PER 1,000) OF DEVELOPING CORONARY

DOES NOT SMOKE CIGARETTES

NO ENLARGED HEART BY ECG

	SBP	105	120	135	150	165	180	195
	Chol.							
GLUCOSE	185	20	24	29	34	40	48	57
INTOLERANCE	210	26	31	37	44	52	61	72
ABSENT	235	34	40	48	56	66	78	92
	260	43	51	61	72	84	99	116
	285	56	66	78	91	107	125	146
	310	71	84	98	115	135	157	181
	335	90	106	124	145	168	194	223

	SBP	105	120	135	150	165	180	195
	Chol.							
GLUCOSE	185	26	30	36	43	50	60	70
INTOLERANCE	210	33	39	46	55	65	76	90
PRESENT	235	42	50	59	70	82	97	113
	260	54	64	75	89	104	122	142
	285	69	82	96	112	131	153	177
	310	88	103	121	141	164	190	218
	335	111	130	151	176	203	233	266

ECG SHOWS ENLARGED HEART (LVH)

	SBP	105	120	135	150	165	180	195
	Chol.							
GLUCOSE	185	34	40	48	56	66	78	92
INTOLERANCE	210	43	51	61	72	84	99	116
ABSENT	235	56	66	78	91	107	125	146
	260	71	84	98	115	135	157	181
	285	90	106	124	145	168	194	223
	310	114	134	155	180	208	238	272
	335	144	167	193	222	254	289	326

	SBP	105	120	135	150	165	180	195
	Chol.							
GLUCOSE	185	42	50	59	70	82	97	113
INTOLERANCE	210	54	64	75	89	104	122	142
PRESENT	235	69	82	96	112	131	153	177
	260	88	103	121	141	164	190	218
	285	111	130	151	176	203	233	266
	310	140	163	188	217	248	283	320
	335	174	201	231	264	300	339	379

*Framingham men aged 45 years have an average SBP of 131 mm. Hg and an average serum cholesterol of 234 mg.%; 68% smoke cigarettes, 0.7% have definite LVH by ECG, and 3.9%

SMOKES CIGARETTES

NO ENLARGED HEART BY ECG

SBP Chol.	105	120	135	150	165	180	195
185	31	37	44	52	61	72	85
210	40	48	56	66	78	92	108
235	52	61	72	85	99	116	136
260	66	78	91	107	125	146	169
285	84	98	115	135	157	181	209
310	106	124	145	168	194	224	256
335	134	155	180	208	238	272	308

SBP Chol.	105	120	135	150	165	180	195
185	39	46	55	65	76	90	105
210	50	59	70	82	97	113	132
235	64	76	89	104	122	142	165
260	82	96	112	131	153	177	204
285	103	121	141	164	190	218	250
310	130	152	176	203	233	266	302
335	163	188	217	248	283	320	360

ECG SHOWS ENLARGED HEART (LVH)

SBP Chol.	105	120	135	150	165	180	195
185	52	61	72	85	99	116	136
210	66	78	91	107	125	146	169
235	84	98	115	135	157	182	209
260	106	124	145	168	194	224	256
285	134	155	180	208	238	272	308
310	167	193	222	254	289	327	367
335	206	237	270	307	345	386	429

SBP Chol.	105	120	135	150	165	180	195
185	64	76	89	104	122	142	165
210	82	96	112	131	153	177	204
235	103	121	141	164	190	218	250
260	130	152	176	203	233	266	302
285	163	188	217	248	283	320	360
310	201	231	264	300	339	379	422
335	247	281	318	358	399	442	486

have glucose intolerance. At these average values the probability of developing coronary heart disease in eight years is 60/1000.

TABLE 1D. PROBABILITY (PER 1,000) OF DEVELOPING CORONARY

NO ENLARGED HEART BY ECG

	SBP	105	120	135	150	165	180	195
	Chol.							
GLUCOSE	185	33	39	46	54	64	75	89
INTOLERANCE	210	40	47	56	66	78	92	107
ABSENT	235	49	58	68	81	95	111	130
	260	60	71	83	98	115	134	156
	285	73	86	101	119	139	161	186
	310	89	105	123	143	166	192	221
	335	108	127	148	171	198	228	260

	SBP	105	120	135	150	165	180	195
	Chol.							
GLUCOSE	185	41	48	57	67	79	93	109
INTOLERANCE	210	50	59	70	82	96	113	132
PRESENT	235	61	72	85	100	117	136	158
	260	75	88	103	121	141	163	189
	285	91	106	125	145	169	195	224
	310	110	129	150	174	201	231	264
	335	133	155	179	207	237	271	307

ECG SHOWS ENLARGED HEART (LVH)

	SBP	105	120	135	150	165	180	195
	Chol.							
GLUCOSE	185	54	63	75	88	103	121	141
INTOLERANCE	210	66	77	91	107	125	145	169
ABSENT	235	80	94	110	129	150	174	201
	260	97	114	133	155	179	207	238
	285	118	137	160	185	213	244	279
	310	142	165	191	220	251	286	324
	335	170	197	226	259	294	332	372

	SBP	105	120	135	150	165	180	195
	Chol.							
GLUCOSE	185	67	78	92	108	127	147	171
INTOLERANCE	210	81	95	112	131	152	176	204
PRESENT	235	99	116	135	157	182	210	241
	260	120	139	162	188	216	248	282
	285	144	167	193	223	255	290	327
	310	173	199	229	262	297	336	376
	335	205	236	269	305	344	385	428

*Framingham men aged 50 years have an average SBP of 133 mm. Hg and an average serum cholesterol of 236 mg.%; 62% smoke cigarettes, 1.5% have definite LVH by ECG, and 6.5%

SMOKES CIGARETTES

NO ENLARGED HEART BY ECG

SBP	105	120	135	150	165	180	195
Chol.							
185	50	59	69	81	96	112	131
210	61	72	84	99	116	135	157
235	74	87	102	120	140	162	188
260	90	106	124	144	168	194	223
285	109	128	149	173	200	229	262
310	132	154	178	206	236	270	306
335	159	184	212	243	277	314	353

SBP	105	120	135	150	165	180	195
Chol.							
185	62	73	86	100	118	137	160
210	75	89	104	122	142	165	191
235	92	107	126	146	170	196	226
260	111	130	151	175	202	232	265
285	134	156	181	208	239	273	309
310	161	186	215	246	280	317	357
335	192	221	253	288	326	366	408

ECG SHOWS ENLARGED HEART (LVH)

SBP	105	120	135	150	165	180	195
Chol.							
185	81	95	111	130	151	175	203
210	98	115	134	156	181	209	239
235	119	139	161	187	215	246	281
260	143	166	192	221	253	288	326
285	172	198	228	260	296	334	375
310	204	235	268	304	343	383	426
335	241	275	312	351	392	435	479

SBP	105	120	135	150	165	180	195
Chol.							
185	100	117	136	158	183	211	242
210	121	141	163	189	218	249	284
235	145	169	195	224	257	292	330
260	174	201	231	264	300	338	379
285	207	238	271	307	346	387	430
310	244	279	315	355	396	439	483
335	286	324	363	405	449	493	537

have glucose intolerance. At these average values the probability of developing coronary heart disease in eight years is 89/1000.

TABLE 1E. PROBABILITY (PER 1,000) OF DEVELOPING CORONARY

DOES NOT SMOKE CIGARETTES

NO ENLARGED HEART BY ECG

	SBP	105	120	135	150	165	180	195
	Chol.							
GLUCOSE	185	46	55	65	76	90	105	123
INTOLERANCE	210	54	64	76	89	105	122	143
ABSENT	235	64	75	88	104	121	142	164
	260	75	88	103	120	140	163	189
	285	87	102	119	139	162	187	216
	310	101	119	138	161	186	214	246
	335	118	137	160	185	213	244	278

	SBP	105	120	135	150	165	180	195
	Chol.							
GLUCOSE	185	58	68	80	94	111	129	151
INTOLERANCE	210	68	80	94	110	128	149	173
PRESENT	235	79	93	109	127	148	172	199
	260	92	108	126	147	171	197	227
	285	107	125	146	170	196	225	258
	310	124	145	168	194	224	256	291
	335	144	167	193	222	254	289	327

ECG SHOWS ENLARGED HEART (LVH)

	SBP	105	120	135	150	165	180	195
	Chol.							
GLUCOSE	185	76	89	105	122	143	166	192
INTOLERANCE	210	88	104	121	142	164	190	219
ABSENT	235	103	120	140	163	189	217	249
	260	119	139	162	187	216	247	282
	285	138	161	186	214	246	280	317
	310	160	185	213	244	278	315	354
	335	183	211	242	276	313	352	394

	SBP	105	120	135	150	165	180	195
	Chol.							
GLUCOSE	185	94	110	128	149	173	200	230
INTOLERANCE	210	109	127	148	172	199	228	261
PRESENT	235	126	147	171	197	227	259	295
	260	146	169	196	225	258	293	331
	285	168	194	224	256	291	329	369
	310	193	222	254	289	327	367	409
	335	221	253	287	325	365	407	450

*Framingham men aged 55 years have an average SBP of 137 mm. Hg and an average serum cholesterol of 234 mg.%; 60% smoke cigarettes, 1.3% have definite LVH by ECG, and 6.2%

SMOKES CIGARETTES

NO ENLARGED HEART BY ECG

SBP	105	120	135	150	165	180	195
Chol.							
185	70	83	97	114	133	155	179
210	82	96	113	132	153	178	205
235	95	112	131	152	176	204	234
260	111	130	151	175	202	232	265
285	129	150	174	201	231	264	299
310	149	173	199	229	262	297	336
335	171	198	228	260	296	334	374

SBP	105	120	135	150	165	180	195
Chol.							
185	87	102	119	139	162	187	216
210	101	118	138	161	186	214	245
235	117	137	159	184	213	244	278
260	136	158	183	211	242	276	313
285	157	182	210	240	274	311	350
310	180	208	239	272	309	348	389
335	207	237	271	307	346	387	430

ECG SHOWS ENLARGED HEART (LVH)

SBP	105	120	135	150	165	180	195
Chol.							
185	113	132	153	178	205	235	269
210	131	152	176	204	234	267	303
235	151	175	202	232	265	301	340
260	174	201	231	264	299	338	378
285	199	229	262	297	336	376	419
310	227	260	296	334	374	416	460
335	258	294	332	372	414	458	502

SBP	105	120	135	150	165	180	195
Chol.							
185	138	161	186	214	245	280	317
210	159	184	213	244	278	315	354
235	183	211	242	276	313	352	393
260	210	240	274	311	350	391	434
285	239	272	309	348	389	432	476
310	271	307	346	387	430	473	518
335	305	344	385	427	471	515	559

have glucose intolerance. At these average values the probability of developing coronary heart disease in eight years is 116/1000.

TABLE 1F. PROBABILITY (PER 1,000) OF DEVELOPING CORONARY

DOES NOT SMOKE CIGARETTES

NO ENLARGED HEART BY ECG

	SBP	105	120	135	150	165	180	195
	Chol.							
GLUCOSE	185	59	70	82	97	113	132	154
INTOLERANCE	210	66	78	92	108	126	147	171
ABSENT	235	74	88	103	120	140	163	189
	260	83	98	114	134	156	180	208
	285	93	109	127	148	172	199	229
	310	104	121	142	164	190	219	251
	335	116	135	157	182	210	240	274

	SBP	105	120	135	150	165	180	195
	Chol.							
GLUCOSE	185	74	87	102	119	139	161	187
INTOLERANCE	210	82	97	113	132	154	179	206
PRESENT	235	92	108	126	147	171	197	227
	260	103	120	140	163	188	217	249
	285	114	134	155	180	208	238	272
	310	127	148	172	199	228	261	297
	335	141	164	190	219	251	285	323

ECG SHOWS ENLARGED HEART (LVH)

	SBP	105	120	135	150	165	180	195
	Chol.							
GLUCOSE	185	96	112	131	153	177	205	235
INTOLERANCE	210	107	125	146	169	196	225	258
ABSENT	235	119	139	162	187	216	247	281
	260	133	154	179	206	237	270	307
	285	147	171	197	227	260	295	333
	310	163	189	217	249	284	321	361
	335	180	208	239	272	309	348	389

	SBP	105	120	135	150	165	180	195
	Chol.							
GLUCOSE	185	118	138	160	185	214	245	279
INTOLERANCE	210	131	153	177	204	235	268	304
PRESENT	235	146	169	196	225	257	293	330
	260	162	187	215	247	281	318	358
	285	179	206	237	270	306	345	386
	310	197	227	259	295	333	373	415
	335	217	249	283	321	360	402	445

*Framingham men aged 60 years have an average SBP of 140 mm. Hg and an average serum cholesterol of 234 mg.%; 50% smoke cigarettes, 1.8% have definite LVH by ECG, and 7.1%

SMOKES CIGARETTES

NO ENLARGED HEART BY ECG

SBP	105	120	135	150	165	180	195
Chol.							
185	89	104	122	143	166	191	220
210	99	116	136	158	183	211	242
235	111	129	151	175	202	232	265
260	123	144	167	193	222	254	289
285	137	159	185	213	244	278	315
310	152	176	204	234	267	303	342
335	169	195	224	256	291	329	370

SBP	105	120	135	150	165	180	195
Chol.							
185	110	128	149	173	200	230	263
210	122	142	165	191	220	252	287
235	136	158	183	211	242	276	312
260	151	175	202	232	265	301	339
285	167	193	222	254	289	327	367
310	184	213	244	278	315	354	395
335	203	234	267	303	341	382	425

ECG SHOWS ENLARGED HEART (LVH)

SBP	105	120	135	150	165	180	195
Chol.							
185	141	164	190	219	251	285	323
210	157	182	209	240	274	311	350
235	174	200	230	263	299	337	378
260	192	221	253	287	325	365	407
285	211	242	276	313	352	394	437
310	232	265	301	340	380	423	467
335	255	290	327	367	409	453	497

SBP	105	120	135	150	165	180	195
Chol.							
185	172	199	228	261	296	335	375
210	190	219	250	285	322	362	404
235	209	240	274	310	350	391	434
260	230	263	299	337	378	420	464
285	252	287	325	365	407	450	494
310	276	313	352	393	436	480	524
335	301	339	380	423	466	511	555

have glucose intolerance. At these average values the probability of developing coronary heart disease in eight years is 134/1000.

TABLE 1G. PROBABILITY (PER 1,000) OF DEVELOPING CORONARY

DOES NOT SMOKE CIGARETTES

NO ENLARGED HEART BY ECG

	SBP	105	120	135	150	165	180	195
	Chol.							
GLUCOSE	185	68	80	94	111	129	150	174
INTOLERANCE	210	73	86	101	118	138	160	186
ABSENT	235	78	92	108	126	147	171	197
	260	84	99	115	135	157	182	209
	285	90	105	123	144	167	193	222
	310	96	113	132	153	178	205	235
	335	103	120	140	163	189	217	249

	SBP	105	120	135	150	165	180	195
	Chol.							
GLUCOSE	185	84	99	116	135	158	182	210
INTOLERANCE	210	90	106	124	144	168	194	223
PRESENT	235	97	113	132	154	178	206	236
	260	103	121	141	164	190	218	250
	285	111	129	151	175	202	232	265
	310	118	138	160	186	214	245	279
	335	126	147	171	197	227	259	295

ECG SHOWS ENLARGED HEART (LVH)

	SBP	105	120	135	150	165	180	195
	Chol.							
GLUCOSE	185	110	128	149	173	200	230	263
INTOLERANCE	210	117	137	159	184	212	243	277
ABSENT	235	125	146	169	196	225	258	293
	260	134	156	180	208	238	272	309
	285	143	166	192	220	252	287	325
	310	152	176	203	234	267	303	341
	335	162	187	216	247	282	319	359

	SBP	105	120	135	150	165	180	195
	Chol.							
GLUCOSE	185	134	156	181	209	240	273	310
INTOLERANCE	210	143	166	193	222	254	288	326
PRESENT	235	153	177	204	235	268	304	343
	260	163	188	217	248	283	320	360
	285	173	200	230	263	298	337	377
	310	184	212	244	278	314	354	395
	335	196	235	258	293	331	371	413

*Framingham men aged 65 years have an average SBP of 141 mm. Hg and an average serum cholesterol of 239 mg.%; 44% smoke cigarettes, 1.4% have definite LVH by ECG, and 8.1%

SMOKES CIGARETTES

NO ENLARGED HEART BY ECG

SBP	105	120	135	150	165	180	195
Chol.							
185	102	119	139	162	187	215	247
210	109	127	148	172	199	228	261
235	116	136	158	183	211	242	276
260	124	145	168	195	224	256	291
285	133	154	179	207	237	271	307
310	142	165	190	219	251	286	323
335	151	175	202	232	265	301	340

SBP	105	120	135	150	165	180	195
Chol.							
185	125	146	169	195	225	257	292
210	133	155	180	208	238	272	308
235	142	165	191	220	252	287	324
260	152	176	203	233	266	302	341
285	162	187	216	247	281	319	358
310	172	199	229	261	297	335	376
335	183	211	242	276	313	352	393

ECG SHOWS ENLARGED HEART (LVH)

SBP	105	120	135	150	165	180	195
Chol.							
185	160	186	214	245	279	316	356
210	171	197	227	259	295	333	373
235	182	209	240	274	311	350	391
260	193	222	254	289	327	367	409
285	205	235	269	305	341	385	427
310	218	249	284	321	361	403	446
335	231	263	299	338	378	421	464

SBP	105	120	135	150	165	180	195
Chol.							
185	194	223	255	290	328	368	410
210	206	237	270	306	345	386	429
235	219	250	285	322	362	404	447
260	232	265	301	339	380	422	466
285	245	280	317	356	398	441	485
310	259	295	333	373	416	459	503
335	274	311	350	391	434	478	522

have glucose intolerance. At these average values the probability of developing coronary heart disease in eight years is 141/1000.

TABLE 1H. PROBABILITY (PER 1,000) OF DEVELOPING CORONARY

DOES NOT SMOKE CIGARETTES

NO ENLARGED HEART BY ECG

	SBP	105	120	135	150	165	180	195
	Chol.							
GLUCOSE	185	71	83	98	114	133	155	180
INTOLERANCE	210	72	85	100	117	137	159	184
ABSENT	235	74	87	103	120	140	163	189
	260	76	90	105	123	144	167	193
	285	78	92	108	126	147	171	197
	310	80	95	111	130	151	175	202
	335	83	97	114	133	155	179	207

	SBP	105	120	135	150	165	180	195
	Chol.							
GLUCOSE	185	87	102	120	140	163	188	217
INTOLERANCE	210	90	105	123	143	166	193	222
PRESENT	235	92	108	126	147	170	197	226
	260	94	111	129	151	175	202	232
	285	97	113	132	154	179	206	237
	310	99	116	136	158	183	211	242
	335	102	119	139	162	187	216	247

ECG SHOWS ENLARGED HEART (LVH)

	SBP	105	120	135	150	165	180	195
	Chol.							
GLUCOSE	185	113	132	154	179	206	237	270
INTOLERANCE	210	116	136	158	183	211	242	276
ABSENT	235	119	139	162	187	216	247	281
	260	122	143	166	192	220	252	287
	285	125	146	170	196	225	258	293
	310	129	150	174	201	230	263	299
	335	132	153	178	205	236	269	305

	SBP	105	120	135	150	165	180	195
	Chol.							
GLUCOSE	185	139	161	187	215	246	281	318
INTOLERANCE	210	142	165	191	220	252	287	324
PRESENT	235	146	169	196	225	257	293	330
	260	149	173	200	230	263	298	337
	285	153	177	205	235	268	304	343
	310	157	182	209	240	274	311	350
	335	161	186	214	245	280	317	356

*Framingham men aged 70 years have an average SBP of 145 mm. Hg and an average serum cholesterol of 231 mg.%; 37% smoke cigarettes, 4.0% have definite LVH by ECG, and 15.2%

SMOKES CIGARETTES

NO ENLARGED HEART BY ECG

SBP	105	120	135	150	165	180	195
Chol.							
185	105	123	144	167	193	222	254
210	108	126	147	171	197	227	259
235	111	129	151	175	202	232	265
260	114	133	154	179	207	237	271
285	117	136	158	183	211	242	276
310	120	139	162	188	216	248	282
335	123	143	166	192	221	253	288

SBP	105	120	135	150	165	180	195
Chol.							
185	129	150	174	201	231	264	300
210	132	154	179	206	237	270	306
235	136	158	183	211	242	276	312
260	139	162	187	216	247	281	318
285	143	166	192	220	252	287	325
310	146	170	196	225	258	293	331
335	150	174	201	230	263	299	337

ECG SHOWS ENLARGED HEART (LVH)

SBP	105	120	135	150	165	180	195
Chol.							
185	165	191	220	252	287	325	365
210	169	196	225	258	293	331	371
235	174	200	230	263	299	337	378
260	178	205	235	269	305	344	385
285	182	210	241	271	311	350	391
310	186	215	246	280	317	357	398
335	191	219	251	286	323	363	405

SBP	105	120	135	150	165	180	195
Chol.							
185	200	230	263	298	337	377	420
210	205	235	268	304	343	384	427
235	209	240	274	310	349	391	434
260	214	245	280	317	356	398	441
285	219	251	285	323	363	404	448
310	224	256	291	329	369	411	455
335	229	262	297	335	376	418	462

have glucose intolerance. At these average values the probability of developing coronary heart disease in eight years is 138/1000.

TABLE 1I. PROBABILITY (PER 1,000) OF DEVELOPING CORONARY

DOES NOT SMOKE CIGARETTES

NO ENLARGED HEART BY ECG

	SBP	105	120	135	150	165	180	195
	Chol.							
GLUCOSE	185	2	2	3	3	4	5	6
INTOLERANCE	210	2	3	4	4	5	7	8
ABSENT	235	3	4	5	6	7	9	10
	260	4	5	6	8	9	11	14
	285	5	7	8	10	12	14	18
	310	7	9	10	13	15	19	23
	335	9	11	13	16	20	24	29

	SBP	105	120	135	150	165	180	195
	Chol.							
GLUCOSE	185	3	4	5	6	7	9	11
INTOLERANCE	210	4	5	6	8	9	11	14
PRESENT	235	6	7	8	10	12	15	18
	260	7	9	11	13	16	19	23
	285	9	11	14	17	21	25	30
	310	12	15	18	22	27	32	39
	335	16	19	23	28	34	42	50

ECG SHOWS ENLARGED HEART (LVH)

	SBP	105	120	135	150	165	180	195
	Chol.							
GLUCOSE	185	4	5	6	7	9	10	13
INTOLERANCE	210	5	6	7	9	11	13	16
ABSENT	235	7	8	10	12	14	17	21
	260	8	10	13	15	19	23	27
	285	11	13	16	20	24	29	35
	310	14	17	21	26	31	38	45
	335	19	23	27	33	40	48	58

	SBP	105	120	135	150	165	180	195
	Chol.							
GLUCOSE	185	7	8	10	12	15	18	22
INTOLERANCE	210	9	11	13	16	19	23	28
PRESENT	235	11	14	17	20	25	30	36
	260	15	18	22	26	32	39	47
	285	19	23	28	34	41	50	60
	310	25	30	36	44	53	64	77
	335	32	39	47	57	68	82	98

*Framingham women aged 35 years have an average SBP of 118 mm. Hg and an average serum cholesterol of 201 mg.%; 56% smoke cigarettes, 0.6% have definite LVH by ECG, and 1.0%

SMOKES CIGARETTES

NO ENLARGED HEART BY ECG

SBP Chol.	105	120	135	150	165	180	195
185	2	2	2	3	3	4	5
210	2	3	3	4	5	6	7
235	3	3	4	5	6	7	9
260	3	4	5	6	8	9	11
285	5	6	7	8	10	12	15
310	6	7	9	11	13	16	19
335	8	9	11	14	17	20	25

SBP Chol.	105	120	135	150	165	180	195
185	3	3	4	5	6	7	9
210	4	4	5	6	8	10	12
235	5	6	7	8	10	12	15
260	6	7	9	11	13	16	20
285	8	10	12	14	17	21	25
310	10	12	15	18	22	27	33
335	13	16	20	24	29	35	42

ECG SHOWS ENLARGED HEART (LVH)

SBP Chol.	105	120	135	150	165	180	195
185	3	4	5	6	7	9	11
210	4	5	6	8	9	11	14
235	5	7	8	10	12	15	18
260	7	9	11	13	16	19	23
285	9	11	14	17	20	25	30
310	12	15	18	22	26	32	38
335	16	19	23	28	34	41	49

SBP Chol.	105	120	135	150	165	180	195
185	6	7	8	10	12	15	18
210	7	9	11	13	16	20	24
235	10	12	14	17	21	25	31
260	12	15	18	22	27	33	40
285	16	20	24	29	35	42	51
310	21	25	31	37	45	54	65
335	27	33	40	48	58	69	83

have glucose intolerance. At these average values the probability of developing coronary heart disease in eight years is 2/1000.

TABLE 1J. PROBABILITY (PER 1,000) OF DEVELOPING CORONARY

DOES NOT SMOKE CIGARETTES

NO ENLARGED HEART BY ECG

	SBP	105	120	135	150	165	180	195
	Chol.							
GLUCOSE	185	4	5	6	8	9	11	14
INTOLERANCE	210	5	6	8	10	12	14	17
ABSENT	235	7	8	10	12	15	18	22
	260	8	10	13	15	19	22	27
	285	11	13	16	19	23	28	34
	310	13	16	20	24	29	35	43
	335	17	21	25	30	37	44	54

	SBP	105	120	135	150	165	180	195
	Chol.							
GLUCOSE	185	7	9	11	13	16	19	24
INTOLERANCE	210	9	11	14	17	20	25	30
PRESENT	235	12	14	17	21	25	31	37
	260	15	18	22	26	32	39	47
	285	19	23	27	33	40	48	58
	310	23	28	34	42	50	61	73
	335	29	36	43	52	63	75	90

ECG SHOWS ENLARGED HEART (LVH)

	SBP	105	120	135	150	165	180	195
	Chol.							
GLUCOSE	185	9	10	13	15	19	23	28
INTOLERANCE	210	11	13	16	19	24	29	35
ABSENT	235	14	17	20	24	30	36	43
	260	17	21	25	31	37	45	54
	285	22	26	32	39	47	56	68
	310	27	33	40	48	58	70	84
	335	34	41	50	60	73	87	104

	SBP	105	120	135	150	165	180	195
	Chol.							
GLUCOSE	185	15	18	22	27	32	39	47
INTOLERANCE	210	19	23	28	34	41	49	59
PRESENT	235	24	29	35	42	51	61	74
	260	30	36	44	53	63	76	91
	285	37	45	55	66	79	95	113
	310	47	56	68	82	98	117	139
	335	58	70	84	101	121	143	169

*Framingham women aged 40 years have an average SBP of 123 mm. Hg and an average serum
cholesterol of 213 mg.%; 53% smoke cigarettes, 0.1% have definite LVH by ECG, and 1.1%

SMOKES CIGARETTES

NO ENLARGED HEART BY ECG

SBP Chol.	105	120	135	150	165	180	195
185	4	4	5	6	8	9	11
210	4	5	7	8	10	12	14
235	6	7	8	10	12	15	18
260	7	9	11	13	16	19	23
285	9	11	13	16	20	24	29
310	11	14	17	20	25	30	36
335	14	17	21	26	31	37	45

SBP Chol.	105	120	135	150	165	180	195
185	6	7	9	11	13	16	20
210	8	9	11	14	17	21	25
235	10	12	14	18	21	26	31
260	12	15	18	22	27	33	39
285	16	19	23	28	34	41	49
310	20	24	29	35	42	51	62
335	25	30	36	44	53	64	77

ECG SHOWS ENLARGED HEART (LVH)

SBP Chol.	105	120	135	150	165	180	195
185	7	9	11	13	16	19	23
210	9	11	13	16	20	24	29
235	11	14	17	21	25	30	37
260	14	18	21	26	31	38	46
285	18	22	27	33	39	48	57
310	23	28	34	41	49	59	71
335	29	35	42	51	62	74	89

SBP Chol.	105	120	135	150	165	180	195
185	13	15	19	22	27	33	40
210	16	19	23	28	34	41	50
235	20	24	29	35	43	52	62
260	25	30	37	44	54	65	78
285	31	38	46	56	67	80	96
310	39	48	58	69	83	100	119
335	49	60	72	86	103	123	146

have glucose intolerance. At these average values the probability of developing coronary heart disease in eight years is 6/1000.

TABLE 1K. PROBABILITY (PER 1,000) OF DEVELOPING CORONARY

DOES NOT SMOKE CIGARETTES

NO ENLARGED HEART BY ECG

	SBP	105	120	135	150	165	180	195
	Chol.							
GLUCOSE	185	8	10	12	15	18	22	27
INTOLERANCE	210	10	12	15	18	22	27	33
ABSENT	235	12	15	18	22	27	33	40
	260	15	19	23	27	33	40	49
	285	19	23	28	33	40	49	59
	310	23	28	34	41	49	59	72
	335	28	34	41	50	60	72	87

	SBP	105	120	135	150	165	180	195
	Chol.							
GLUCOSE	185	14	18	21	26	31	38	46
INTOLERANCE	210	18	21	26	32	38	46	56
PRESENT	235	22	26	32	39	47	56	68
	260	27	32	39	47	57	68	82
	285	32	39	47	57	69	83	99
	310	40	48	58	69	83	100	119
	335	48	58	70	84	100	120	142

ECG SHOWS ENLARGED HEART (LVH)

	SBP	105	120	135	150	165	180	195
	Chol.							
GLUCOSE	185	17	21	25	30	37	44	53
INTOLERANCE	210	21	25	30	37	45	54	65
ABSENT	235	25	31	37	45	54	65	78
	260	31	37	45	55	66	79	95
	285	38	46	55	66	80	95	114
	310	46	56	67	80	96	115	137
	335	56	67	81	97	116	138	163

	SBP	105	120	135	150	165	180	195
	Chol.							
GLUCOSE	185	29	35	43	52	62	75	90
INTOLERANCE	210	36	43	52	63	75	91	108
PRESENT	235	43	52	63	76	91	109	130
	260	53	64	77	92	110	131	155
	285	64	77	93	111	132	156	184
	310	78	93	111	133	157	185	217
	335	94	112	134	158	186	218	254

*Framingham women aged 45 years have an average SBP of 129 mm. Hg and an average serum cholesterol of 228 mg.%; 52% smoke cigarettes, 0.4% have definite LVH by ECG, and 2.7%

SMOKES CIGARETTES

NO ENLARGED HEART BY ECG

SBP	105	120	135	150	165	180	195
Chol.							
185	7	8	10	13	15	19	22
210	9	10	13	15	19	23	27
235	10	13	15	19	23	28	34
260	13	16	19	23	28	34	41
285	16	19	23	28	34	41	50
310	19	23	28	34	42	50	61
335	24	29	35	42	51	61	73

SBP	105	120	135	150	165	180	195
Chol.							
185	12	15	18	22	26	32	39
210	15	18	22	27	32	39	47
235	18	22	27	32	39	48	57
260	22	27	33	40	48	58	70
285	27	33	40	48	58	70	84
310	33	40	49	59	71	85	102
335	41	49	59	71	85	102	122

ECG SHOWS ENLARGED HEART (LVH)

SBP	105	120	135	150	165	180	195
Chol.							
185	14	17	21	25	31	37	45
210	17	21	26	31	38	45	55
235	21	26	31	38	46	55	67
260	26	32	38	46	56	67	81
285	32	38	47	56	68	81	97
310	39	47	57	68	82	98	117
335	47	57	69	82	99	118	140

SBP	105	120	135	150	165	180	195
Chol.							
185	25	30	36	44	53	63	76
210	30	36	44	53	64	77	92
235	37	44	54	64	77	93	111
260	45	54	65	78	94	112	133
285	54	65	79	94	113	134	159
310	66	79	95	113	135	160	188
335	80	96	114	136	161	190	222

have glucose intolerance. At these average values the probability of developing coronary heart disease in eight years is 15/1000.

TABLE 1L. PROBABILITY (PER 1,000) OF DEVELOPING CORONARY

DOES NOT SMOKE CIGARETTES

NO ENLARGED HEART BY ECG

	SBP	105	120	135	150	165	180	195
	Chol.							
GLUCOSE	185	15	18	21	26	32	38	46
INTOLERANCE	210	17	21	26	31	38	45	55
ABSENT	235	21	25	30	37	45	54	65
	260	25	30	36	44	53	64	76
	285	29	35	43	52	62	75	90
	310	35	42	51	61	74	88	106
	335	41	50	60	72	87	104	124

	SBP	105	120	135	150	165	180	195
	Chol.							
GLUCOSE	185	25	31	37	45	54	65	78
INTOLERANCE	210	30	36	44	53	64	77	92
PRESENT	235	36	43	52	63	75	90	108
	260	42	51	62	74	89	106	127
	285	50	60	73	87	104	124	148
	310	59	71	86	102	122	145	171
	335	70	84	101	120	143	168	198

ECG SHOWS ENLARGED HEART (LVH)

	SBP	105	120	135	150	165	180	195
	Chol.							
GLUCOSE	185	29	36	43	52	63	76	91
INTOLERANCE	210	35	42	51	62	74	89	106
ABSENT	235	42	50	60	73	87	104	124
	260	49	59	71	86	103	122	145
	285	58	70	84	101	120	143	169
	310	69	83	99	118	140	166	195
	335	81	97	116	138	163	192	224

	SBP	105	120	135	150	165	180	195
	Chol.							
GLUCOSE	185	50	61	73	88	105	125	148
INTOLERANCE	210	60	72	86	103	123	146	172
PRESENT	235	70	85	101	121	143	170	199
	260	83	99	119	141	167	196	229
	285	98	117	139	164	193	226	262
	310	114	136	161	190	222	258	298
	335	134	158	187	219	254	294	336

*Framingham women aged 50 years have an average SBP of 136 mm. Hg and an average serum cholesterol of 246 mg.%; 41% smoke cigarettes, 0.2% have definite LVH by ECG, and 2.9%

SMOKES CIGARETTES

NO ENLARGED HEART BY ECG

SBP	105	120	135	150	165	180	195
Chol.							
185	12	15	18	22	27	32	39
210	15	18	21	26	32	38	46
235	17	21	26	31	38	45	55
260	21	25	30	37	45	54	65
285	25	30	36	44	53	64	76
310	29	35	43	52	62	75	90
335	35	42	51	61	74	88	106

SBP	105	120	135	150	165	180	195
Chol.							
185	21	26	31	38	46	55	66
210	25	31	37	45	54	65	78
235	30	36	44	53	64	77	92
260	36	43	52	63	75	90	108
285	42	51	62	74	89	106	127
310	50	60	73	87	104	124	147
335	59	71	86	102	122	145	171

ECG SHOWS ENLARGED HEART (LVH)

SBP	105	120	135	150	165	180	195
Chol.							
185	25	30	36	44	53	64	77
210	29	36	43	52	63	75	91
235	35	42	51	62	74	89	106
260	41	50	60	73	87	104	124
285	49	59	71	86	103	122	145
310	58	70	84	101	120	143	169
335	69	83	99	118	140	166	195

SBP	105	120	135	150	165	180	195
Chol.							
185	43	51	62	75	89	107	127
210	50	61	73	88	105	125	148
235	60	72	86	103	123	146	172
260	70	85	101	121	143	169	199
285	83	99	119	141	167	196	229
310	98	117	139	164	193	226	262
335	114	136	161	190	222	258	298

have glucose intolerance. At these average values the probability of developing coronary heart disease in eight years is 31/1000.

TABLE 1M. PROBABILITY (PER 1,000) OF DEVELOPING CORONARY

DOES NOT SMOKE CIGARETTES

NO ENLARGED HEART BY ECG

	SBP	105	120	135	150	165	180	195
	Chol.							
GLUCOSE	185	23	28	33	40	49	59	71
INTOLERANCE	210	26	32	39	47	56	68	81
ABSENT	235	30	37	44	54	65	78	93
	260	35	42	51	62	74	89	107
	285	41	49	59	71	85	102	122
	310	47	56	68	82	98	117	139
	335	54	65	78	93	112	133	157

	SBP	105	120	135	150	165	180	195
	Chol.							
GLUCOSE	185	39	47	57	69	82	99	118
INTOLERANCE	210	45	54	66	79	95	113	134
PRESENT	235	52	63	75	90	108	129	153
	260	60	72	86	103	123	146	173
	285	69	83	99	118	140	166	195
	310	79	95	113	135	159	188	220
	335	91	108	129	153	180	212	246

ECG SHOWS ENLARGED HEART (LVH)

	SBP	105	120	135	150	165	180	195
	Chol.							
GLUCOSE	185	46	55	66	80	95	114	135
INTOLERANCE	210	52	63	76	91	109	130	154
ABSENT	235	60	73	87	104	124	148	174
	260	69	83	100	119	142	167	197
	285	80	96	114	136	161	189	221
	310	91	109	130	154	182	213	248
	335	105	125	148	175	205	239	277

	SBP	105	120	135	150	165	180	195
	Chol.							
GLUCOSE	185	77	92	110	131	156	184	215
INTOLERANCE	210	88	106	126	149	176	207	241
PRESENT	235	101	121	143	169	199	233	270
	260	116	137	163	191	224	260	300
	285	132	156	184	216	251	290	332
	310	150	177	208	242	280	322	366
	335	170	200	233	270	311	355	402

*Framingham women aged 55 years have an average SBP of 142 mm. Hg and an average serum cholesterol of 257 mg.%; 34% smoke cigarettes, 1.5% have definite LVH by ECG, and 4.9%

SMOKES CIGARETTES

NO ENLARGED HEART BY ECG

SBP	105	120	135	150	165	180	195
Chol.							
185	19	23	28	34	41	50	60
210	22	27	32	39	48	57	69
235	26	31	38	45	55	66	79
260	30	36	43	52	63	76	91
285	34	41	50	60	72	87	104
310	39	48	57	69	83	99	119
335	45	55	66	79	95	114	135

SBP	105	120	135	150	165	180	195
Chol.							
185	33	40	48	58	70	84	101
210	38	46	56	67	80	96	115
235	44	53	64	77	92	110	131
260	51	61	73	88	105	126	149
285	58	70	84	101	120	143	169
310	67	81	96	115	137	162	191
335	77	92	110	131	156	183	215

ECG SHOWS ENLARGED HEART (LVH)

SBP	105	120	135	150	165	180	195
Chol.							
185	38	46	56	67	81	97	116
210	44	53	64	77	93	111	132
235	51	62	74	89	106	127	150
260	59	71	85	102	121	144	170
285	68	81	97	116	138	163	192
310	78	93	111	132	157	185	217
335	89	106	127	150	178	208	243

SBP	105	120	135	150	165	180	195
Chol.							
185	65	79	94	112	134	158	187
210	75	90	108	128	152	179	210
235	86	103	123	146	172	202	236
260	99	118	140	165	195	228	264
285	113	134	159	187	219	255	294
310	129	152	180	211	246	284	326
335	146	173	203	237	274	315	360

have glucose intolerance. At these average values the probability of developing coronary heart disease in eight years is 54/1000.

DOES NOT SMOKE CIGARETTES

NO ENLARGED HEART BY ECG

	SBP	105	120	135	150	165	180	195
	Chol.							
GLUCOSE	185	32	38	46	56	67	81	97
INTOLERANCE	210	35	43	52	62	75	90	108
ABSENT	235	40	48	58	70	84	100	120
	260	45	54	65	78	94	112	133
	285	50	60	73	87	104	124	148
	310	56	68	81	97	116	138	163
	335	63	76	91	108	129	153	181

	SBP	105	120	135	150	165	180	195
	Chol.							
GLUCOSE	185	54	65	78	94	112	133	158
INTOLERANCE	210	60	73	87	104	124	148	174
PRESENT	235	68	81	97	116	138	163	192
	260	76	91	108	129	153	181	212
	285	85	101	121	143	169	199	233
	310	94	113	134	159	187	219	255
	335	105	125	149	176	206	240	278

ECG SHOWS ENLARGED HEART (LVH)

	SBP	105	120	135	150	165	180	195
	Chol.							
GLUCOSE	185	63	75	90	108	129	152	180
INTOLERANCE	210	70	84	101	120	143	169	198
ABSENT	235	78	94	112	133	158	186	218
	260	88	105	125	148	175	205	239
	285	98	117	139	164	193	226	262
	310	109	130	154	181	212	247	286
	335	121	144	170	200	233	271	311

	SBP	105	120	135	150	165	180	195
	Chol.							
GLUCOSE	185	105	125	148	175	205	239	277
INTOLERANCE	210	117	139	164	193	226	262	302
PRESENT	235	130	154	181	212	247	286	328
	260	144	170	200	233	271	311	355
	285	159	188	220	256	295	338	383
	310	176	207	241	279	321	365	412
	335	194	227	264	304	348	394	442

*Framingham women aged 60 years have an average SBP of 149 mm. Hg and an average serum cholesterol of 261 mg.%; 26% smoke cigarettes, 2.0% have definite LVH by ECG, and 4.7%

SMOKES CIGARETTES

NO ENLARGED HEART BY ECG

SBP	105	120	135	150	165	180	195
Chol.							
185	27	32	39	47	57	68	82
210	30	36	44	53	64	76	92
235	34	41	49	59	71	85	102
260	38	46	55	66	80	95	114
285	42	51	62	74	89	106	127
310	47	57	69	83	99	118	140
335	53	64	77	92	110	131	156

SBP	105	120	135	150	165	180	195
Chol.							
185	46	55	66	80	95	114	135
210	51	62	74	89	106	127	150
235	57	69	83	99	118	141	166
260	64	77	92	110	131	156	184
285	72	86	103	123	146	172	202
310	80	96	115	136	161	190	223
335	90	107	128	151	178	209	244

ECG SHOWS ENLARGED HEART (LVH)

SBP	105	120	135	150	165	180	195
Chol.							
185	53	64	77	92	110	131	155
210	59	71	86	103	122	145	171
235	66	80	96	114	136	161	189
260	74	89	107	127	151	178	209
285	83	99	119	141	167	196	229
310	93	111	132	156	184	216	251
335	103	123	146	173	203	237	274

SBP	105	120	135	150	165	180	195
Chol.							
185	89	107	127	151	178	209	243
210	99	119	141	167	196	229	266
235	111	132	156	184	216	251	290
260	123	146	173	203	237	275	316
285	137	162	191	223	259	299	342
310	152	179	210	245	283	325	370
335	168	198	231	268	308	352	398

have glucose intolerance. At these average values the probability of developing coronary heart disease in eight years is 77/1000.

TABLE 1O. PROBABILITY (PER 1,000) OF DEVELOPING CORONARY

DOES NOT SMOKE CIGARETTES

NO ENLARGED HEART BY ECG

	SBP	105	120	135	150	165	180	195
	Chol.							
GLUCOSE	185	39	47	57	68	82	98	117
INTOLERANCE	210	43	51	62	75	89	107	127
ABSENT	235	47	56	68	81	97	116	138
	260	51	61	74	88	106	126	149
	285	55	67	80	96	115	136	161
	310	60	73	87	104	124	148	174
	335	66	79	95	113	135	159	188

	SBP	105	120	135	150	165	180	195
	Chol.							
GLUCOSE	185	·66	80	95	114	136	161	189
INTOLERANCE	210	72	87	104	124	147	173	204
PRESENT	235	79	94	113	134	159	187	219
	260	86	102	122	145	171	201	235
	285	93	111	132	157	185	217	252
	310	101	121	143	169	199	233	270
	335	110	131	155	183	214	249	288

ECG SHOWS ENLARGED HEART (LVH)

	SBP	105	120	135	150	165	180	195
	Chol.							
GLUCOSE	185	77	92	110	131	155	183	215
INTOLERANCE	210	84	100	119	142	168	197	230
ABSENT	235	91	109	129	153	181	212	247
	260	99	118	140	166	195	228	265
	285	107	128	152	179	210	245	283
	310	117	139	164	193	226	262	302
	335	126	150	177	208	242	280	322

	SBP	105	120	135	150	165	180	195
	Chol.							
GLUCOSE	185	127	151	178	209	244	282	324
INTOLERANCE	210	138	163	192	225	261	301	344
PRESENT	235	149	176	207	241	279	321	365
	260	161	190	222	258	298	341	387
	285	174	204	238	276	317	362	409
	310	188	220	256	295	338	383	431
	335	202	236	273	314	359	405	454

*Framingham women aged 65 years have an average SBP of 151 mm. Hg and an average serum cholesterol of 269 mg.%; 23% smoke cigarettes, 3.1% have definite LVH by ECG, and 9.0%

SMOKES CIGARETTES

NO ENLARGED HEART BY ECG

SBP	105	120	135	150	165	180	195
Chol.							
185	33	40	48	58	70	84	100
210	36	43	52	63	76	91	109
235	39	47	57	69	83	99	118
260	43	52	62	75	90	108	128
285	47	56	68	82	98	117	139
310	51	62	74	89	106	127	150
335	56	67	81	97	115	137	162

SBP	105	120	135	150	165	180	195
Chol.							
185	56	68	81	97	116	138	163
210	61	74	88	106	126	149	176
235	67	80	96	115	136	161	190
260	73	87	104	124	148	174	205
285	79	95	113	135	159	188	220
310	86	103	123	146	172	202	236
335	94	112	133	158	186	218	253

ECG SHOWS ENLARGED HEART (LVH)

SBP	105	120	135	150	165	180	195
Chol.							
185	65	78	94	112	133	158	186
210	71	85	102	122	144	171	200
235	77	93	111	132	156	184	216
260	84	101	120	143	169	198	232
285	91	109	130	154	182	213	248
310	99	119	141	167	196	229	266
335	108	129	152	180	211	246	284

SBP	105	120	135	150	165	180	195
Chol.							
185	109	129	153	181	212	247	286
210	118	140	166	195	228	265	305
235	128	152	179	210	245	283	325
260	139	164	193	226	262	302	345
285	150	177	208	242	280	322	367
310	162	191	223	259	299	342	388
335	175	205	240	277	319	363	410

have glucose intolerance. At these average values the probability of developing coronary heart disease in eight years is 95/1000.

TABLE 1P. PROBABILITY (PER 1,000) OF DEVELOPING CORONARY

DOES NOT SMOKE CIGARETTES

NO ENLARGED HEART BY ECG

	SBP	105	120	135	150	165	180	195
	Chol.							
GLUCOSE	185	43	52	63	75	90	108	129
INTOLERANCE	210	46	55	67	80	96	114	136
ABSENT	235	49	59	71	85	101	121	144
	260	52	62	75	90	107	128	152
	285	55	66	79	95	114	135	160
	310	58	70	84	101	120	143	169
	335	62	74	89	107	127	151	178

	SBP	105	120	135	150	165	180	195
	Chol.							
GLUCOSE	185	73	88	105	125	148	175	206
INTOLERANCE	210	77	93	111	132	156	184	216
PRESENT	235	82	98	117	140	165	194	227
	260	87	104	124	147	174	204	238
	285	92	110	131	155	183	215	250
	310	98	117	139	164	193	226	262
	335	103	123	146	173	203	237	275

ECG SHOWS ENLARGED HEART (LVH)

	SBP	105	120	135	150	165	180	195
	Chol.							
GLUCOSE	185	85	101	121	143	169	199	233
INTOLERANCE	210	90	107	128	151	179	209	244
ABSENT	235	95	113	135	160	188	220	256
	260	101	120	142	168	198	231	268
	285	106	127	150	177	208	243	281
	310	113	134	159	187	219	255	294
	335	119	141	167	197	230	267	307

	SBP	105	120	135	150	165	180	195
	Chol.							
GLUCOSE	185	139	165	194	227	263	303	347
INTOLERANCE	210	147	174	204	238	276	317	361
PRESENT	235	155	183	214	250	289	331	376
	260	164	193	225	262	302	345	391
	285	173	203	237	274	315	359	406
	310	182	213	248	287	329	374	422
	335	191	224	260	300	343	389	437

*Framingham women aged 70 years have an average SBP of 158 mm. Hg and an average serum cholesterol of 267 mg.%; 15% smoke cigarettes, 1.4% have definite LVH by ECG, and 8.1%

SMOKES CIGARETTES

NO ENLARGED HEART BY ECG

SBP	105	120	135	150	165	180	195
Chol.							
185	36	44	53	64	77	92	110
210	39	47	56	68	81	98	116
235	41	50	60	72	86	103	123
260	44	51	61	76	91	109	130
285	46	56	67	81	97	116	137
310	49	59	71	86	103	122	145
335	52	63	76	91	109	129	153

SBP	105	120	135	150	165	180	195
Chol.							
185	62	74	89	107	127	151	178
210	66	79	95	113	134	159	187
235	70	84	100	119	142	168	197
260	74	89	106	126	150	177	208
285	78	94	112	133	158	186	218
310	83	99	119	141	167	196	229
335	88	105	125	149	176	206	241

ECG SHOWS ENLARGED HEART (LVH)

SBP	105	120	135	150	165	180	195
Chol.							
185	72	86	103	123	146	172	202
210	76	91	109	130	154	182	213
235	81	97	115	137	162	191	224
260	86	102	122	145	171	201	235
285	91	108	129	153	180	212	246
310	96	115	136	161	190	222	258
335	102	121	144	170	200	233	271

SBP	105	120	135	150	165	180	195
Chol.							
185	119	142	167	197	230	267	308
210	126	150	177	207	242	280	321
235	133	158	186	218	253	293	335
260	141	166	196	229	266	306	350
285	149	175	206	240	278	320	364
310	157	185	216	252	291	334	379
335	165	195	227	264	304	348	394

have glucose intolerance. At these average values the probability of developing coronary heart disease in eight years is 103/1000.

APPENDIX 2

TABLE 2.

Cardiovascular Disease

TABLE 2A. PROBABILITY (PER 1,000) OF DEVELOPING CARDIOVASCULAR

DOES NOT SMOKE CIGARETTES

NO ENLARGED HEART BY ECG

	SBP	105	120	135	150	165	180	195
	Chol.							
GLUCOSE	185	6	7	9	11	14	18	23
INTOLERANCE	210	8	10	12	16	20	25	31
ABSENT	235	11	14	17	21	27	34	43
	260	15	19	24	30	37	47	58
	285	20	26	32	41	51	64	79
	310	28	35	44	56	69	86	107
	335	39	49	61	76	94	116	142

	SBP	105	120	135	150	165	180	195
	Chol.							
GLUCOSE	185	10	13	16	20	26	32	40
INTOLERANCE	210	14	18	22	28	35	44	55
PRESENT	235	19	24	31	39	48	60	75
	260	27	34	42	53	66	82	101
	285	37	46	58	72	89	110	135
	310	50	63	78	97	120	147	179
	335	69	85	105	130	159	193	232

ECG SHOWS ENLARGED HEART (LVH)

	SBP	105	120	135	150	165	180	195
	Chol.							
GLUCOSE	185	16	20	25	32	40	50	62
INTOLERANCE	210	22	28	35	43	54	68	84
ABSENT	235	30	38	47	59	74	92	113
	260	41	52	65	80	100	123	150
	285	57	70	88	108	133	163	197
	310	77	95	118	144	176	213	255
	335	104	128	156	190	229	273	322

	SBP	105	120	135	150	165	180	195
	Chol.							
GLUCOSE	185	29	36	45	56	70	87	108
INTOLERANCE	210	39	49	61	76	95	117	144
PRESENT	235	54	67	83	103	127	155	189
	260	73	91	112	138	168	203	244
	285	99	122	149	181	219	262	310
	310	132	161	196	235	280	330	384
	335	174	211	253	300	351	406	464

*Framingham men aged 35 years have an average SBP of 127 mm. Hg and an average serum cholesterol of 220 mg.%; 70% smoke cigarettes, 0.0% have definite LVH by ECG, and 1.7%

SMOKES CIGARETTES

NO ENLARGED HEART BY ECG

SBP	105	120	135	150	165	180	195
Chol.							
185	10	12	15	19	25	31	39
210	13	17	21	27	34	42	53
235	19	23	29	37	46	58	72
260	26	32	40	51	63	79	97
285	35	44	55	69	86	106	130
310	48	60	75	93	115	141	172
335	66	82	101	125	153	186	224

SBP	105	120	135	150	165	180	195
Chol.							
185	18	22	28	35	44	55	69
210	24	31	38	48	60	75	93
235	33	42	52	65	81	101	124
260	46	57	71	89	110	135	165
285	63	78	96	119	146	178	215
310	85	105	129	158	192	231	276
335	114	140	171	207	248	295	346

ECG SHOWS ENLARGED HEART (LVH)

SBP	105	120	135	150	165	180	195
Chol.							
185	27	34	43	54	67	84	104
210	38	47	59	73	91	112	138
235	51	64	80	99	122	150	182
260	70	87	108	132	162	197	236
285	95	117	144	175	212	254	301
310	127	155	189	228	272	321	374
335	168	204	244	290	341	396	453

SBP	105	120	135	150	165	180	195
Chol.							
185	49	61	76	94	116	143	174
210	67	83	102	126	155	188	227
235	90	111	137	167	203	243	289
260	121	148	181	218	261	309	361
285	160	195	234	279	329	383	440
310	210	251	298	350	405	463	522
335	269	318	371	428	486	545	602

have glucose intolerance. At these average values the probability of developing cardiovascular disease in eight years is 18/1000.

DOES NOT SMOKE CIGARETTES

NO ENLARGED HEART BY ECG

	SBP	105	120	135	150	165	180	195
	Chol.							
GLUCOSE	185	12	15	19	23	29	37	46
INTOLERANCE	210	15	19	24	31	39	48	60
ABSENT	235	20	26	32	40	51	63	79
	260	27	34	42	53	66	82	102
	285	35	44	55	69	86	106	131
	310	46	58	72	90	111	136	167
	335	61	76	94	116	142	173	210

	SBP	105	120	135	150	165	180	195
	Chol.							
GLUCOSE	185	21	27	33	42	52	65	81
INTOLERANCE	210	28	35	44	55	68	85	105
PRESENT	235	37	46	57	71	89	110	135
	260	48	60	75	93	115	141	172
	285	63	78	97	119	147	178	216
	310	82	101	125	153	186	224	267
	335	106	130	159	193	232	277	326

ECG SHOWS ENLARGED HEART (LVH)

	SBP	105	120	135	150	165	180	195
	Chol.							
GLUCOSE	185	33	41	51	64	80	99	122
INTOLERANCE	210	43	54	67	83	103	127	156
ABSENT	235	56	70	87	108	133	162	197
	260	73	91	113	138	169	204	245
	285	95	117	144	176	212	254	301
	310	122	150	183	220	264	312	364
	335	156	190	229	273	322	375	432

	SBP	105	120	135	150	165	180	195
	Chol.							
GLUCOSE	185	58	73	90	111	137	167	202
INTOLERANCE	210	76	94	116	143	174	210	252
PRESENT	235	98	121	148	181	218	261	309
	260	126	155	188	227	270	319 ˎ	372
	285	161	195	235	280	330	383	441
	310	203	244	290	340	395	453	511
	335	253	300	351	407	464	523	581

*Framingham men aged 40 years have an average SBP of 129 mm. Hg and an average serum cholesterol of 228 mg.%; 70% smoke cigarettes, 0.3% have definite LVH by ECG, and 3.3%

SMOKES CIGARETTES

NO ENLARGED HEART BY ECG

SBP	105	120	135	150	165	180	195
Chol.							
185	20	25	32	40	50	63	78
210	27	33	42	53	66	82	101
235	35	44	55	69	85	106	130
260	46	58	72	89	110	135	165
285	60	75	93	115	141	172	208
310	78	97	120	147	179	216	259
335	101	125	153	186	225	268	317

SBP	105	120	135	150	165	180	195
Chol.							
185	36	45	57	71	88	109	134
210	48	60	74	92	114	140	170
235	62	77	96	119	145	177	214
260	81	100	124	152	184	222	266
285	105	129	158	192	231	275	325
310	134	164	199	239	285	335	389
335	171	207	248	295	346	401	459

ECG SHOWS ENLARGED HEART (LVH)

SBP	105	120	135	150	165	180	195
Chol.							
185	56	70	86	107	132	161	195
210	73	90	112	137	168	203	244
235	94	117	143	174	211	253	300
260	122	149	181	219	262	310	362
285	155	189	227	271	320	373	430
310	196	236	281	331	385	442	500
335	245	291	341	396	454	512	571

SBP	105	120	135	150	165	180	195
Chol.							
185	97	120	147	180	217	259	307
210	125	154	187	225	269	317	371
235	160	194	234	278	328	382	439
260	202	242	288	339	393	450	509
285	251	298	349	405	462	521	579
310	308	360	416	474	533	591	646
335	371	428	486	545	602	657	708

have glucose intolerance. At these average values the probability of developing cardiovascular disease in eight years is 41/1000.

TABLE 2C. PROBABILITY (PER 1,000) OF DEVELOPING CARDIOVASCULAR

DOES NOT SMOKE CIGARETTES

NO ENLARGED HEART BY ECG

	SBP	105	120	135	150	165	180	195
	Chol.							
GLUCOSE	185	22	27	35	43	54	68	84
INTOLERANCE	210	28	35	43	54	68	84	104
ABSENT	235	35	44	54	68	84	104	129
	260	44	55	68	85	105	129	158
	285	55	68	85	105	129	158	192
	310	68	85	105	130	158	192	232
	335	85	105	130	159	193	232	277

	SBP	105	120	135	150	165	180	195
	Chol.							
GLUCOSE	185	39	49	61	76	95	117	143
INTOLERANCE	210	49	61	76	95	117	144	175
PRESENT	235	62	77	95	117	144	176	212
	260	77	95	118	144	176	213	255
	285	96	118	145	176	213	255	303
	310	118	145	177	214	256	303	355
	335	145	177	214	256	304	356	411

ECG SHOWS ENLARGED HEART (LVH)

	SBP	105	120	135	150	165	180	195
	Chol.							
GLUCOSE	185	60	75	93	115	141	172	208
INTOLERANCE	210	75	93	115	141	172	209	250
ABSENT	235	93	115	142	173	209	251	297
	260	116	142	173	209	251	298	349
	285	142	173	210	252	298	350	405
	310	174	210	252	299	351	406	464
	335	211	253	300	351	406	464	523

	SBP	105	120	135	150	165	180	195
	Chol.							
GLUCOSE	185	105	129	158	191	231	275	324
INTOLERANCE	210	129	158	192	231	275	325	378
PRESENT	235	158	192	232	276	325	379	436
	260	193	232	277	326	380	436	495
	285	232	277	327	380	437	496	554
	310	278	327	381	438	496	555	612
	335	328	382	438	497	556	613	667

*Framingham men aged 45 years have an average SBP of 131 mm. Hg and an average serum cholesterol of 234 mg.%; 68% smoke cigarettes, 0.7% have definite LVH by ECG, and 3.9%

SMOKES CIGARETTES

NO ENLARGED HEART BY ECG

SBP	105	120	135	150	165	180	195
Chol.							
185	38	47	59	73	91	112	138
210	47	59	73	91	113	138	169
235	59	74	91	113	139	169	205
260	74	92	113	139	170	206	247
285	92	113	139	170	206	247	293
310	114	140	170	206	248	294	345
335	140	171	207	248	295	346	401

SBP	105	120	135	150	165	180	195
Chol.							
185	67	83	102	126	154	188	226
210	83	103	126	155	188	227	271
235	103	127	155	189	227	271	320
260	127	156	189	228	272	321	374
285	156	189	228	272	321	375	431
310	190	229	273	322	375	432	490
335	229	273	323	376	433	491	550

ECG SHOWS ENLARGED HEART (LVH)

SBP	105	120	135	150	165	180	195
Chol.							
185	101	124	152	185	223	266	315
210	124	152	185	223	267	315	368
235	153	186	224	267	316	369	425
260	186	224	268	316	369	426	484
285	225	268	317	370	426	485	543
310	269	318	371	427	485	544	602
335	318	371	428	486	545	602	657

SBP	105	120	135	150	165	180	195
Chol.							
185	170	205	246	293	344	399	456
210	206	247	293	344	399	457	516
235	247	294	345	400	457	516	574
260	294	346	400	458	517	575	631
285	346	401	459	518	576	632	685
310	402	459	518	576	633	685	734
335	460	519	577	633	686	734	778

have glucose intolerance. At these average values the probability of developing coronary heart disease in eight years is 75/1000.

TABLE 2D. PROBABILITY (PER 1,000) OF DEVELOPING CARDIOVASCULAR

DOES NOT SMOKE CIGARETTES

NO ENLARGED HEART BY ECG

	SBP	105	120	135	150	165	180	195
	Chol.							
GLUCOSE	185	37	46	57	71	89	110	135
INTOLERANCE	210	44	55	69	85	106	130	159
ABSENT	235	53	66	82	102	125	153	187
	260	63	79	98	121	148	180	218
	285	76	94	116	143	174	211	252
	310	91	112	138	168	204	244	290
	335	108	133	162	197	237	282	332

	SBP	105	120	135	150	165	180	195
	Chol.							
GLUCOSE	185	65	81	100	123	151	184	222
INTOLERANCE	210	78	96	119	146	177	214	257
PRESENT	235	93	114	140	171	207	249	295
	260	110	135	165	200	241	286	337
	285	130	160	194	233	278	327	381
	310	154	187	226	269	318	371	428
	335	181	218	261	309	361	417	475

ECG SHOWS ENLARGED HEART (LVH)

	SBP	105	120	135	150	165	180	195
	Chol.							
GLUCOSE	185	98	121	148	181	218	261	309
INTOLERANCE	210	117	143	175	211	253	300	352
ABSENT	235	138	169	204	245	291	342	397
	260	163	197	237	282	332	387	444
	285	191	230	274	323	377	433	492
	310	222	266	314	367	423	481	540
	335	257	305	357	412	470	529	587

	SBP	105	120	135	150	165	180	195
	Chol.							
GLUCOSE	185	166	201	241	287	338	392	449
INTOLERANCE	210	194	234	279	328	382	439	498
PRESENT	235	226	270	319	372	429	487	546
	260	262	310	362	418	476	535	593
	285	301	352	408	466	524	583	638
	310	343	398	455	514	572	629	682
	335	387	445	503	562	619	672	722

*Framingham men aged 50 years have an average SBP of 133 mm. Hg and an average serum cholesterol of 236 mg.%; 62% smoke cigarettes, 1.5% have definite LVH by ECG, and 6.5%

SMOKES CIGARETTES

NO ENLARGED HEART BY ECG

SBP	105	120	135	150	165	180	195
Chol.							
185	62	78	96	119	146	177	214
210	75	92	114	140	171	207	249
235	89	110	135	165	200	241	286
260	106	130	159	194	233	278	327
285	126	154	187	225	269	318	371
310	148	181	218	261	309	361	417
335	174	211	253	300	351	407	465

SBP	105	120	135	150	165	180	195
Chol.							
185	108	133	163	197	237	282	332
210	128	157	191	230	274	323	376
235	151	184	222	265	314	367	423
260	178	215	257	305	357	412	470
285	208	249	296	347	402	460	519
310	241	287	337	392	449	508	566
335	278	328	382	439	497	556	613

ECG SHOWS ENLARGED HEART (LVH)

SBP	105	120	135	150	165	180	195
Chol.							
185	160	194	234	278	328	382	439
210	188	226	270	319	372	428	487
235	219	262	309	362	418	476	535
260	253	300	352	408	465	524	582
285	292	343	397	455	514	572	628
310	333	387	444	503	561	618	672
335	377	434	492	551	608	663	713

SBP	105	120	135	150	165	180	195
Chol.							
185	258	305	358	413	471	530	588
210	296	348	403	461	519	578	634
235	338	393	450	509	567	624	677
260	383	440	498	557	614	668	718
285	429	487	546	604	658	709	755
310	477	536	593	649	700	747	789
335	525	583	639	691	739	782	819

have glucose intolerance. At these average values the probability of developing cardiovascular disease in eight years is 115/1000.

TABLE 2E. PROBABILITY (PER 1,000) OF DEVELOPING CARDIOVASCULAR

DOES NOT SMOKE CIGARETTES

NO ENLARGED HEART BY ECG

	SBP	105	120	135	150	165	180	195
	Chol.							
GLUCOSE	185	55	69	85	105	130	159	193
INTOLERANCE	210	63	79	97	120	147	179	217
ABSENT	235	72	90	111	137	167	202	243
	260	83	103	127	155	188	227	271
	285	95	117	144	175	212	254	301
	310	108	133	163	198	238	283	333
	335	124	151	184	222	266	314	367

	SBP	105	120	135	150	165	180	195
	Chol.							
GLUCOSE	185	96	118	145	177	214	256	304
INTOLERANCE	210	110	135	165	200	240	285	336
PRESENT	235	125	153	186	224	268	316	369
	260	142	173	209	251	209	349	404
	285	161	195	235	280	330	383	440
	310	182	219	262	310	363	419	477
	335	205	246	292	343	398	455	514

ECG SHOWS ENLARGED HEART (LVH)

	SBP	105	120	135	150	165	180	195
	Chol.							
GLUCOSE	185	143	174	211	252	299	351	406
INTOLERANCE	210	162	196	236	281	331	385	442
ABSENT	235	183	221	264	312	365	421	479
	260	206	247	294	345	400	457	516
	285	231	276	325	379	436	494	553
	310	259	306	358	414	472	531	589
	335	288	338	393	450	509	567	624

	SBP	105	120	135	150	165	180	195
	Chol.							
GLUCOSE	185	233	278	328	381	438	497	556
INTOLERANCE	210	261	309	361	417	475	534	592
PRESENT	235	290	341	396	453	512	570	627
	260	322	375	431	490	549	606	661
	285	355	410	468	527	585	641	693
	310	389	446	505	563	620	674	723
	335	425	483	542	599	654	705	752

*Framingham men aged 55 years have an average SBP of 137 mm. Hg and an average serum cholesterol of 234 mg.%; 60% smoke cigarettes, 1.3% have definite LVH by ECG, and 6.2%

SMOKES CIGARETTES

NO ENLARGED HEART BY ECG

SBP	105	120	135	150	165	180	195
Chol.							
185	92	114	140	171	207	248	294
210	105	130	159	193	232	277	326
235	120	147	179	217	259	307	359
260	137	167	202	243	289	339	394
285	155	188	227	271	320	373	430
310	175	212	254	301	353	408	466
335	198	238	283	333	387	444	503

SBP	105	120	135	150	165	180	195
Chol.							
185	157	190	229	273	322	376	432
210	177	214	256	304	356	411	469
235	200	240	285	336	390	447	506
260	224	268	316	369	426	484	543
285	251	298	349	404	462	521	579
310	280	329	383	440	499	558	615
335	310	363	419	477	536	594	649

ECG SHOWS ENLARGED HEART (LVH)

SBP	105	120	135	150	165	180	195
Chol.							
185	226	269	318	371	428	486	545
210	252	299	351	406	464	523	581
235	281	331	385	442	501	559	616
260	312	365	421	479	538	595	651
285	345	400	457	516	574	631	683
310	379	435	494	553	610	664	715
335	414	472	531	589	644	696	744

SBP	105	120	135	150	165	180	195
Chol.							
185	347	402	460	519	577	633	686
210	381	438	497	555	613	667	717
235	417	475	534	592	647	699	746
260	453	512	570	627	680	729	773
285	490	549	606	661	711	757	798
310	527	585	641	693	741	783	820
335	563	620	674	723	768	807	841

have glucose intolerance. At these average values the probability of developing cardiovascular disease in eight years is 159/1000.

TABLE 2F. PROBABILITY (PER 1,000) OF DEVELOPING CARDIOVASCULAR

DOES NOT SMOKE CIGARETTES

NO ENLARGED HEART BY ECG

	SBP	105	120	135	150	165	180	195
	Chol.							
GLUCOSE	185	74	92	114	140	170	206	247
INTOLERANCE	210	81	101	124	152	185	224	267
ABSENT	235	89	111	136	166	201	242	288
	260	98	121	148	181	218	261	309
	285	108	132	162	196	236	281	331
	310	118	145	176	213	255	302	354
	335	129	158	192	231	275	325	378

	SBP	105	120	135	150	165	180	195
	Chol.							
GLUCOSE	185	128	156	190	229	273	322	375
INTOLERANCE	210	139	170	206	247	293	345	399
PRESENT	235	152	185	223	267	315	368	424
	260	166	201	241	287	338	392	449
	285	180	218	261	309	361	417	475
	310	196	236	281	331	385	442	500
	335	213	255	302	354	409	467	526

ECG SHOWS ENLARGED HEART (LVH)

	SBP	105	120	135	150	165	180	195
	Chol.							
GLUCOSE	185	187	225	269	317	371	427	485
INTOLERANCE	210	203	243	289	340	395	452	511
ABSENT	235	220	263	311	363	419	478	536
	260	238	283	333	387	445	503	562
	285	257	304	356	412	470	529	587
	310	277	326	380	437	495	554	611
	335	298	349	405	462	521	579	635

	SBP	105	120	135	150	165	180	195
	Chol.							
GLUCOSE	185	295	347	402	459	518	576	632
INTOLERANCE	210	317	370	426	485	543	601	656
PRESENT	235	340	394	452	510	569	625	679
	260	363	419	477	536	594	649	701
	285	387	444	503	561	618	672	722
	310	412	469	528	586	642	694	742
	335	437	495	554	611	665	715	761

*Framingham men aged 60 years have an average SBP of 140 mm. Hg and an average serum
cholesterol of 234 mg.%; 50% smoke cigarettes, 1.8% have definite LVH by ECG, and 7.1%

SMOKES CIGARETTES

NO ENLARGED HEART BY ECG

SBP Chol.	105	120	135	150	165	180	195
185	123	150	183	221	264	312	365
210	134	164	199	239	284	335	389
235	147	179	216	258	306	358	414
260	160	194	234	278	328	382	439
285	174	211	252	299	351	406	464
310	189	228	272	321	375	431	490
335	206	247	293	344	399	456	515

SBP Chol.	105	120	135	150	165	180	195
185	204	244	290	341	396	453	512
210	221	264	312	365	421	479	538
235	239	284	334	389	446	504	563
260	258	305	357	413	471	530	588
285	278	328	381	438	497	555	612
310	299	350	406	464	522	580	637
335	321	374	431	489	548	605	660

ECG SHOWS ENLARGED HEART (LVH)

SBP Chol.	105	120	135	150	165	180	195
185	286	337	391	448	507	566	622
210	308	360	416	474	533	591	646
235	330	384	441	499	558	615	669
260	353	408	466	525	583	639	691
285	377	433	492	550	608	662	713
310	401	459	517	576	632	685	733
335	426	484	543	600	655	706	753

SBP Chol.	105	120	135	150	165	180	195
185	423	481	540	597	653	704	750
210	448	507	565	622	675	725	769
235	473	532	590	646	697	745	787
260	499	558	615	669	719	764	804
285	525	583	639	691	739	782	819
310	550	607	662	712	758	799	834
335	575	631	684	733	776	815	848

have glucose intolerance. At these average values the probability of developing cardiovascular disease in eight years is 193/1000.

TABLE 2G. PROBABILITY (PER 1,000) OF DEVELOPING CARDIOVASCULAR

DOES NOT SMOKE CIGARETTES

NO ENLARGED HEART BY ECG

	SBP	105	120	135	150	165	180	195
	Chol.							
GLUCOSE	185	90	112	137	167	203	244	289
INTOLERANCE	210	95	117	144	175	212	254	301
ABSENT	235	100	123	151	184	222	265	314
	260	105	130	159	193	232	276	326
	285	111	136	166	202	242	288	339
	310	117	143	175	211	253	300	352
	335	123	150	183	221	264	312	365

	SBP	105	120	135	150	165	180	195
	Chol.							
GLUCOSE	185	153	186	225	268	317	370	427
INTOLERANCE	210	161	195	235	280	330	384	441
PRESENT	235	169	204	245	292	342	397	455
	260	177	214	256	303	355	411	469
	285	185	224	267	316	369	425	483
	310	194	234	279	328	382	439	497
	335	203	244	290	341	396	453	512

ECG SHOWS ENLARGED HEART (LVH)

	SBP	105	120	135	150	165	180	195
	Chol.							
GLUCOSE	185	221	265	313	366	422	480	539
INTOLERANCE	210	231	276	325	379	436	494	553
ABSENT	235	242	287	338	392	450	508	567
	260	252	299	351	406	464	523	581
	285	263	311	364	420	478	537	595
	310	275	324	377	434	492	551	608
	335	286	336	391	448	507	565	622

	SBP	105	120	135	150	165	180	195
	Chol.							
GLUCOSE	185	342	396	454	513	571	628	681
INTOLERANCE	210	355	410	468	527	585	641	693
PRESENT	235	368	424	482	541	599	654	705
	260	381	438	497	555	612	667	717
	285	395	452	511	569	626	679	728
	310	409	466	525	583	639	692	739
	335	422	481	539	597	652	704	750

*Framingham men aged 65 years have an average SBP of 141 mm. Hg and an average serum cholesterol of 239 mg.%; 44% smoke cigarettes, 1.4% have definite LVH by ECG, and 8.1%

SMOKES CIGARETTES

NO ENLARGED HEART BY ECG

SBP	105	120	135	150	165	180	195
Chol.							
185	148	180	217	260	308	360	416
210	155	189	227	271	320	373	430
235	163	197	237	283	333	387	444
260	171	207	248	294	345	400	458
285	179	216	259	306	358	414	472
310	187	226	270	319	372	428	487
335	196	236	281	331	385	442	501

SBP	105	120	135	150	165	180	195
Chol.							
185	240	286	336	391	448	507	565
210	251	298	349	404	462	521	579
235	262	310	362	418	476	535	593
260	273	322	376	432	491	549	607
285	285	335	389	446	505	564	620
310	296	348	403	461	519	578	634
335	308	361	417	475	534	591	647

ECG SHOWS ENLARGED HEART (LVH)

SBP	105	120	135	150	165	180	195
Chol.							
185	332	386	443	502	560	617	671
210	345	400	457	516	574	631	684
235	358	413	471	530	588	644	696
260	371	427	486	544	602	657	708
285	384	441	500	559	616	670	719
310	398	456	514	573	629	682	731
335	412	470	529	587	642	694	742

SBP	105	120	135	150	165	180	195
Chol.							
185	476	534	592	648	699	746	788
210	490	549	606	661	711	757	798
235	504	563	620	673	723	767	807
260	519	577	633	686	734	778	816
285	533	591	646	698	745	787	824
310	547	604	659	710	756	797	832
335	561	618	672	722	766	806	840

have glucose intolerance. At these average values the probability of developing cardiovascular disease in eight years is 212/1000.

TABLE 2H. PROBABILITY (PER 1,000) OF DEVELOPING CARDIOVASCULAR

DOES NOT SMOKE CIGARETTES

NO ENLARGED HEART BY ECG

	SBP	105	120	135	150	165	180	195
	Chol.							
GLUCOSE	185	100	123	150	183	221	264	312
INTOLERANCE	210	101	124	152	185	223	266	.315
ABSENT	235	102	125	153	187	225	269	317
	260	103	127	155	188	227	271	320
	285	104	128	157	190	229	273	323
	310	105	129	158	192	231	276	325
	335	106	131	160	194	233	278	328

	SBP	105	120	135	150	165	180	195
	Chol.							
GLUCOSE	185	168	203	244	290	341	396	453
INTOLERANCE	210	170	205	246	293	344	399	456
PRESENT	235	171	207	249	295	346	401	459
	260	173	209	251	298	349	404	462
	285	175	211	253	300	352	407	465
	310	176	213	255	303	355	410	468
	335	178	215	258	305	357	413	471

ECG SHOWS ENLARGED HEART (LVH)

	SBP	105	120	135	150	165	180	195
	Chol.							
GLUCOSE	185	241	286	337	391	448	507	565
INTOLERANCE	210	243	289	339	394	451	510	568
ABSENT	235	245	291	342	397	454	513	571
	260	247	294	345	400	457	516	574
	285	249	296	347	402	460	519	577
	310	252	299	350	405	463	522	580
	335	254	301	353	408	466	525	583

	SBP	105	120	135	150	165	180	195
	Chol.							
GLUCOSE	185	366	423	481	540	597	652	704
INTOLERANCE	210	369	426	484	543	600	655	706
PRESENT	235	372	428	487	546	603	658	709
	260	375	431	490	549	606	661	711
	285	378	434	493	551	609	663	714
	310	380	437	496	554	612	666	716
	335	383	440	499	557	614	668	718

*Framingham men aged 70 years have an average SBP of 145 mm. Hg and an average serum cholesterol of 231 mg.%; 37% smoke cigarettes, 4.0% have definite LVH by ECG, and 15.2%

SMOKES CIGARETTES

NO ENLARGED HEART BY ECG

SBP / Chol.	105	120	135	150	165	180	195
185	162	196	236	281	331	385	442
210	164	198	238	284	334	388	445
235	165	200	241	286	337	391	448
260	167	202	243	289	339	394	451
285	168	204	245	291	342	397	454
310	170	206	247	294	345	400	457
335	172	208	249	296	347	402	460

SBP / Chol.	105	120	135	150	165	180	195
185	261	309	361	417	475	534	592
210	263	311	364	420	478	537	594
235	265	314	366	423	481	540	597
260	268	316	369	426	484	543	600
285	270	319	372	428	487	546	603
310	272	321	375	431	490	549	606
335	275	324	378	434	493	551	609

ECG SHOWS ENLARGED HEART (LVH)

SBP / Chol.	105	120	135	150	165	180	195
185	356	412	470	529	587	642	695
210	359	415	473	532	590	645	697
235	362	418	476	535	593	648	700
260	365	421	479	538	595	651	702
285	367	424	482	541	598	653	705
310	370	427	485	544	601	656	707
335	373	429	488	547	604	659	710

SBP / Chol.	105	120	135	150	165	180	195
185	503	561	618	672	722	766	806
210	506	564	621	675	724	769	808
235	509	567	624	677	726	771	810
260	512	570	627	680	729	773	811
285	515	573	629	682	731	775	813
310	518	576	632	685	733	777	815
335	521	579	635	688	736	779	817

have glucose intolerance. At these average values the probability of developing cardiovascular disease in eight years is 229/1000.

TABLE 2I. PROBABILITY (PER 1,000) OF DEVELOPING CARDIOVASCULAR

DOES NOT SMOKE CIGARETTES

NO ENLARGED HEART BY ECG

	SBP	105	120	135	150	165	180	195
	Chol.							
GLUCOSE	185	4	5	6	7	9	11	13
INTOLERANCE	210	5	6	7	9	11	13	17
ABSENT	235	6	7	9	11	13	17	20
	260	7	9	11	13	17	20	25
	285	9	11	13	16	20	25	31
	310	11	13	16	20	25	31	38
	335	13	16	20	25	31	38	47

	SBP	105	120	135	150	165	180	195
	Chol.							
GLUCOSE	185	7	9	11	14	17	21	26
INTOLERANCE	210	9	11	14	17	21	26	32
PRESENT	235	11	14	17	21	26	32	40
	260	14	17	21	26	32	40	49
	285	17	21	26	32	39	49	60
	310	21	26	32	39	48	59	73
	335	26	32	39	48	59	72	88

ECG SHOWS ENLARGED HEART (LVH)

	SBP	105	120	135	150	165	180	195
	Chol.							
GLUCOSE	185	9	11	14	17	21	26	32
INTOLERANCE	210	11	14	17	21	26	32	39
ABSENT	235	14	17	21	26	32	39	48
	260	17	21	25	31	39	48	58
	285	21	25	31	39	47	58	71
	310	25	31	38	47	58	71	87
	335	31	38	47	58	71	86	105

	SBP	105	120	135	150	165	180	195
	Chol.							
GLUCOSE	185	17	21	27	33	40	50	61
INTOLERANCE	210	21	26	33	40	49	61	74
PRESENT	235	26	33	40	49	60	74	90
	260	32	40	49	60	74	90	109
	285	40	49	60	73	90	109	132
	310	49	60	73	89	109	131	158
	335	60	73	89	108	131	158	189

*Framingham women aged 35 years have an average SBP of 118 mm. Hg and an average serum cholesterol of 201 mg.%; 56% smoke cigarettes, 0.6% have definite LVH by ECG, and 1.0%

SMOKES CIGARETTES

NO ENLARGED HEART BY ECG

SBP Chol.	105	120	135	150	165	180	195
185	4	5	6	7	9	11	14
210	5	6	7	9	11	14	17
235	6	7	9	11	14	17	21
260	7	9	11	14	17	21	26
285	9	11	14	17	21	26	32
310	11	14	17	21	26	32	40
335	14	17	21	26	32	39	48

SBP Chol.	105	120	135	150	165	180	195
185	8	9	12	14	18	22	27
210	9	12	14	18	22	27	34
235	12	14	18	22	27	34	41
260	14	18	22	27	33	41	51
285	18	22	27	33	41	50	62
310	22	27	33	41	50	62	75
335	27	33	41	50	61	75	92

ECG SHOWS ENLARGED HEART (LVH)

SBP Chol.	105	120	135	150	165	180	195
185	9	11	14	18	22	27	33
210	11	14	17	22	27	33	40
235	14	17	21	27	33	40	50
260	17	21	26	33	40	49	61
285	21	26	33	40	49	60	74
310	26	32	40	49	60	74	90
335	32	40	49	60	73	90	109

SBP Chol.	105	120	135	150	165	180	195
185	18	22	28	34	42	52	63
210	22	27	34	42	51	63	77
235	27	34	42	51	63	77	94
260	34	41	51	63	76	93	113
285	41	51	62	76	93	113	136
310	51	62	76	93	112	136	163
335	62	76	92	112	136	163	195

have glucose intolerance. At these average values the probability of developing cardiovascular disease in eight years is 5/1000.

TABLE 2J. PROBABILITY (PER 1,000) OF DEVELOPING CARDIOVASCULAR

DOES NOT SMOKE CIGARETTES

NO ENLARGED HEART BY ECG

	SBP	105	120	135	150	165	180	195
	Chol.							
GLUCOSE	185	7	9	11	14	17	21	26
INTOLERANCE	210	9	11	13	16	20	25	31
ABSENT	235	10	13	16	20	24	30	37
	260	12	15	19	24	29	36	44
	285	15	18	23	28	35	43	53
	310	18	22	27	34	42	51	63
	335	22	27	33	40	50	61	75

	SBP	105	120	135	150	165	180	195
	Chol.							
GLUCOSE	185	14	17	22	27	33	40	50
INTOLERANCE	210	17	21	26	32	39	48	59
PRESENT	235	20	25	31	38	47	58	70
	260	24	30	37	45	56	68	84
	285	29	36	44	54	67	81	99
	310	35	43	53	65	79	96	117
	335	42	51	63	77	94	114	137

ECG SHOWS ENLARGED HEART (LVH)

	SBP	105	120	135	150	165	180	195
	Chol.							
GLUCOSE	185	17	21	26	32	39	49	60
INTOLERANCE	210	20	25	31	38	47	58	71
ABSENT	235	24	30	37	46	56	69	84
	260	29	36	44	55	67	82	100
	285	35	43	53	65	80	97	118
	310	42	52	63	77	94	114	138
	335	50	61	75	92	111	135	162

	SBP	105	120	135	150	165	180	195
	Chol.							
GLUCOSE	185	33	41	50	61	75	92	111
INTOLERANCE	210	40	49	60	73	89	108	131
PRESENT	235	47	58	71	87	105	128	154
	260	56	69	84	103	124	150	179
	285	67	82	100	121	146	175	208
	310	80	97	118	142	171	203	241
	335	94	115	138	166	199	235	276

*Framingham women aged 40 years have an average SBP of 123 mm. Hg and an average serum cholesterol of 213 mg.%; 53% smoke cigarettes, 0.1% have definite LVH by ECG, and 1.1%

SMOKES CIGARETTES

NO ENLARGED HEART BY ECG

SBP	105	120	135	150	165	180	195
Chol.							
185	7	9	11	14	18	22	27
210	9	11	14	17	21	26	32
235	11	13	16	20	25	31	38
260	13	16	20	24	30	37	46
285	16	19	24	29	36	44	55
310	19	23	28	35	43	53	65
335	22	28	34	42	52	63	77

SBP	105	120	135	150	165	180	195
Chol.							
185	15	18	22	28	34	42	52
210	18	22	27	33	41	50	61
235	21	26	32	40	49	60	73
260	25	31	38	47	58	71	87
285	30	37	46	56	69	84	103
310	36	45	55	67	82	100	121
335	43	53	65	80	97	118	142

ECG SHOWS ENLARGED HEART (LVH)

SBP	105	120	135	150	165	180	195
Chol.							
185	18	22	27	33	41	50	62
210	21	26	32	40	49	60	74
235	25	31	39	48	58	71	87
260	30	38	46	57	69	85	103
285	36	45	55	67	82	100	122
310	44	54	66	80	98	118	143
335	52	64	78	95	115	139	167

SBP	105	120	135	150	165	180	195
Chol.							
185	34	42	52	64	78	95	115
210	41	51	62	76	92	112	136
235	49	60	74	90	109	132	159
260	58	72	87	106	129	155	185
285	70	85	103	125	151	181	215
310	83	101	122	147	176	210	248
335	98	119	143	172	205	242	284

have glucose intolerance. At these average values the probability of developing cardiovascular disease in eight years is 12/1000.

DOES NOT SMOKE CIGARETTES

NO ENLARGED HEART BY ECG

	SBP	105	120	135	150	165	180	195
	Chol.							
GLUCOSE	185	13	16	20	24	30	37	46
INTOLERANCE	210	15	19	23	29	35	43	53
ABSENT	235	18	22	27	33	41	50	62
	260	21	25	31	39	48	59	72
	285	24	30	37	45	55	68	83
	310	28	35	43	52	64	79	96
	335	33	40	50	61	75	91	111

	SBP	105	120	135	150	165	180	195
	Chol.							
GLUCOSE	185	25	31	38	47	58	71	87
INTOLERANCE	210	29	36	45	55	67	82	100
PRESENT	235	34	42	52	64	78	95	115
	260	40	49	60	74	90	109	132
	285	47	57	70	85	104	126	152
	310	54	66	81	99	120	144	173
	335	63	77	94	114	138	165	197

ECG SHOWS ENLARGED HEART (LVH)

	SBP	105	120	135	150	165	180	195
	Chol.							
GLUCOSE	185	30	37	46	57	69	85	103
INTOLERANCE	210	35	44	54	66	80	98	119
ABSENT	235	41	51	62	76	93	113	136
	260	48	59	72	88	107	130	156
	285	56	68	84	102	123	149	178
	310	65	79	97	117	142	170	203
	335	75	92	111	135	162	194	230

	SBP	105	120	135	150	165	180	195
	Chol.							
GLUCOSE	185	58	72	87	106	128	155	185
INTOLERANCE	210	68	83	101	122	147	177	210
PRESENT	235	79	96	116	140	168	201	238
	260	91	110	133	160	192	228	268
	285	105	127	153	183	218	257	300
	310	121	146	175	208	246	288	335
	335	139	166	199	235	277	322	371

*Framingham women aged 45 years have an average SBP of 129 mm. Hg and an average serum cholesterol of 228 mg.%; 52% smoke cigarettes, 0.4% have definite LVH by ECG, and 2.7%

SMOKES CIGARETTES

NO ENLARGED HEART BY ECG

SBP	105	120	135	150	165	180	195
Chol.							
185	13	17	21	25	31	39	47
210	16	19	24	30	37	45	55
235	18	23	28	35	43	52	64
260	21	26	33	40	49	61	74
285	25	31	38	47	58	70	86
310	29	36	44	54	67	82	99
335	34	42	52	63	77	94	114

SBP	105	120	135	150	165	180	195
Chol.							
185	26	32	40	49	60	74	90
210	31	38	46	57	70	85	104
235	36	44	54	66	81	98	119
260	42	51	63	77	93	113	137
285	48	59	73	89	108	130	157
310	56	69	84	102	124	149	179
335	65	80	97	118	142	171	204

ECG SHOWS ENLARGED HEART (LVH)

SBP	105	120	135	150	165	180	195
Chol.							
185	32	39	48	59	72	88	107
210	37	45	56	68	83	101	123
235	43	53	65	79	96	117	141
260	50	61	75	91	111	134	161
285	58	71	87	105	128	154	184
310	67	82	100	121	146	176	209
335	78	95	115	139	167	200	237

SBP	105	120	135	150	165	180	195
Chol.							
185	61	74	90	110	133	160	191
210	70	86	104	126	152	182	217
235	81	99	120	145	174	207	245
260	94	114	138	166	198	235	276
285	109	131	158	189	224	264	309
310	125	151	180	215	253	296	343
335	143	172	205	243	285	331	380

have glucose intolerance. At these average values the probability of developing cardiovascular disease in eight years is 25/1000.

TABLE 2L. PROBABILITY (PER 1,000) OF DEVELOPING CARDIOVASCULAR

DOES NOT SMOKE CIGARETTES

NO ENLARGED HEART BY ECG

	SBP	105	120	135	150	165	180	195
	Chol.							
GLUCOSE	185	22	27	33	41	50	62	75
INTOLERANCE	210	25	31	38	46	57	70	85
ABSENT	235	28	35	43	53	64	79	96
	260	32	39	49	60	73	89	108
	285	36	45	55	67	82	100	121
	310	41	51	62	76	93	113	136
	335	47	57	70	86	105	127	153

	SBP	105	120	135	150	165	180	195
	Chol.							
GLUCOSE	185	42	52	64	78	95	115	139
INTOLERANCE	210	48	59	72	88	107	129	155
PRESENT	235	54	66	81	99	120	145	174
	260	61	75	92	111	135	162	193
	285	69	85	103	125	151	180	215
	310	78	96	116	140	168	201	238
	335	89	108	130	157	188	223	263

ECG SHOWS ENLARGED HEART (LVH)

	SBP	105	120	135	150	165	180	195
	Chol.							
GLUCOSE	185	51	62	76	93	113	136	164
INTOLERANCE	210	57	70	86	104	126	152	182
ABSENT	235	65	79	97	117	142	170	203
	260	73	90	109	132	159	190	225
	285	83	101	122	148	177	211	249
	310	94	114	137	165	197	233	274
	335	105	128	154	184	219	258	301

	SBP	105	120	135	150	165	180	195
	Chol.							
GLUCOSE	185	96	116	140	168	201	238	279
INTOLERANCE	210	108	130	157	187	223	262	306
PRESENT	235	121	146	175	208	246	289	335
	260	136	163	195	231	272	316	365
	285	152	182	216	255	298	346	396
	310	170	202	239	281	327	376	428
	335	189	224	264	308	356	407	460

*Framingham women aged 50 years have an average SBP of 136 mm. Hg and an average serum cholesterol of 246 mg.%; 41% smoke cigarettes, 0.2% have definite LVH by ECG, and 2.9%

SMOKES CIGARETTES

NO ENLARGED HEART BY ECG

SBP	105	120	135	150	165	180	195
Chol.							
185	23	28	34	42	52	64	78
210	26	32	39	48	59	72	88
235	29	36	44	55	67	82	99
260	33	41	50	62	76	92	112
285	38	46	57	70	85	104	126
310	43	53	65	79	96	117	141
335	49	60	73	89	108	131	158

SBP	105	120	135	150	165	180	195
Chol.							
185	44	54	66	81	98	119	144
210	50	61	75	91	111	134	161
235	56	69	84	102	124	150	179
260	64	78	95	115	139	167	200
285	77	88	107	129	156	186	221
310	81	99	120	145	174	207	245
335	92	112	135	162	194	230	270

ECG SHOWS ENLARGED HEART (LVH)

SBP	105	120	135	150	165	180	195
Chol.							
185	53	65	79	96	117	141	169
210	60	73	89	108	131	158	188
235	67	82	100	122	147	176	209
260	76	93	113	136	164	196	232
285	86	105	127	153	183	217	256
310	97	118	142	171	203	241	282
335	109	132	159	190	226	266	310

SBP	105	120	135	150	165	180	195
Chol.							
185	99	120	145	174	207	245	287
210	111	135	162	194	230	270	315
235	125	151	181	215	254	297	344
260	140	168	201	238	279	325	374
285	157	188	223	263	307	355	405
310	175	209	247	289	335	385	438
335	195	231	272	317	365	417	470

have glucose intolerance. At these average values the probability of developing cardiovascular disease in eight years is 48/1000.

TABLE 2M. PROBABILITY (PER 1,000) OF DEVELOPING CARDIOVASCULAR

DOES NOT SMOKE CIGARETTES

NO ENLARGED HEART BY ECG

	SBP	105	120	135	150	165	180	195
	Chol.							
GLUCOSE	185	34	42	52	64	78	95	115
INTOLERANCE	210	38	47	57	70	86	104	126
ABSENT	235	42	52	63	78	94	115	139
	260	46	57	70	85	104	126	152
	285	51	63	77	94	114	138	166
	310	57	69	85	103	125	151	181
	335	63	77	93	113	137	165	197

	SBP	105	120	135	150	165	180	195
	Chol.							
GLUCOSE	185	66	80	98	119	143	172	205
INTOLERANCE	210	73	88	108	130	157	187	223
PRESENT	235	80	97	118	143	171	204	241
	260	88	107	129	156	186	222	261
	285	97	117	142	170	203	240	282
	310	106	129	155	185	220	260	304
	335	117	141	169	202	239	280	326

ECG SHOWS ENLARGED HEART (LVH)

	SBP	105	120	135	150	165	180	195
	Chol.							
GLUCOSE	185	79	96	116	140	169	201	238
INTOLERANCE	210	87	105	127	154	184	219	258
ABSENT	235	95	116	140	168	200	237	278
	260	105	127	153	183	217	256	300
	285	115	139	167	199	236	277	322
	310	126	152	182	216	255	298	346
	335	138	166	198	235	276	321	370

	SBP	105	120	135	150	165	180	195
	Chol.							
GLUCOSE	185	144	173	206	244	286	332	382
INTOLERANCE	210	158	189	224	264	308	356	407
PRESENT	235	172	205	243	285	331	381	433
	260	188	223	263	307	355	406	459
	285	204	242	284	330	379	431	485
	310	222	262	305	353	404	457	511
	335	241	282	328	377	429	483	537

*Framingham women aged 55 years have an average SBP of 142 mm. Hg and an average serum cholesterol of 257 mg.%; 34% smoke cigarettes, 1.5% have definite LVH by ECG, and 4.9%

SMOKES CIGARETTES

NO ENLARGED HEART BY ECG

SBP	105	120	135	150	165	180	195
Chol.							
185	36	44	54	66	81	98	119
210	39	49	60	73	89	108	131
235	44	54	66	80	98	119	143
260	48	59	73	88	108	130	157
285	53	65	80	97	118	143	171
310	59	72	88	107	129	156	186
335	65	79	97	117	142	170	203

SBP	105	120	135	150	165	180	195
Chol.							
185	68	83	101	123	148	178	212
210	75	92	111	135	162	194	230
235	83	101	122	147	177	210	249
260	91	111	134	161	193	228	269
285	100	122	147	176	209	247	290
310	110	133	160	191	227	267	312
335	121	146	175	208	246	289	335

ECG SHOWS ENLARGED HEART (LVH)

SBP	105	120	135	150	165	180	195
Chol.							
185	82	99	120	145	174	208	245
210	90	109	132	159	190	225	265
235	99	120	144	173	206	244	286
260	108	131	158	189	224	264	308
285	119	144	172	205	243	285	331
310	130	157	188	223	263	307	355
335	143	171	204	242	284	330	379

SBP	105	120	135	150	165	180	195
Chol.							
185	149	179	213	252	294	341	391
210	163	195	231	272	317	365	417
235	178	212	250	293	340	390	442
260	194	230	271	315	364	415	468
285	211	249	292	338	388	441	495
310	229	269	314	362	414	467	521
335	248	290	337	387	439	493	547

have glucose intolerance. At these average values the probability of developing cardiovascular disease in eight years is 80/1000.

DOES NOT SMOKE CIGARETTES

NO ENLARGED HEART BY ECG

	SBP	105	120	135	150	165	180	195
	Chol.							
GLUCOSE	185	51	62	76	93	113	136	164
INTOLERANCE	210	55	67	82	99	121	146	175
ABSENT	235	59	72	88	107	129	155	186
	260	63	77	94	114	138	166	198
	285	68	83	101	122	148	177	211
	310	73	89	108	131	158	189	224
	335	79	96	116	140	168	201	238

	SBP	105	120	135	150	165	180	195
	Chol.							
GLUCOSE	185	96	116	140	168	201	238	279
INTOLERANCE	210	102	124	150	179	213	252	295
PRESENT	235	110	133	160	191	227	267	311
	260	118	142	171	203	241	283	328
	285	126	152	182	216	255	299	346
	310	135	162	194	230	270	315	364
	335	144	173	206	244	286	332	382

ECG SHOWS ENLARGED HEART (LVH)

	SBP	105	120	135	150	165	180	195
	Chol.							
GLUCOSE	185	113	137	165	197	233	274	319
INTOLERANCE	210	122	147	176	209	248	290	336
ABSENT	235	130	157	187	223	262	306	354
	260	139	167	200	236	278	323	372
	285	149	178	212	251	294	340	390
	310	159	190	226	266	310	358	409
	335	170	202	240	281	327	376	428

	SBP	105	120	135	150	165	180	195
	Chol.							
GLUCOSE	185	202	239	281	326	376	428	481
INTOLERANCE	210	215	254	297	344	393	447	501
PRESENT	235	228	269	313	362	413	466	520
	260	242	284	330	380	432	486	540
	285	257	300	348	398	451	505	559
	310	272	317	366	417	471	525	578
	335	288	334	384	436	490	544	597

*Framingham women aged 60 years have an average SBP of 149 mm. Hg and an average serum cholesterol of 261 mg.%; 26% smoke cigarettes, 2.0% have definite LVH by ECG, and 4.7%

SMOKES CIGARETTES

NO ENLARGED HEART BY ECG

SBP	105	120	135	150	165	180	195
Chol.							
185	53	65	79	96	117	141	169
210	57	69	85	103	125	151	180
235	61	75	91	111	134	161	192
260	66	80	98	118	143	172	205
285	71	86	105	127	153	183	217
310	76	92	112	136	163	195	231
335	81	99	120	145	174	207	245

SBP	105	120	135	150	165	180	195
Chol.							
185	99	120	145	174	207	245	287
210	106	129	155	185	220	260	303
235	114	138	165	197	234	275	320
260	122	147	176	210	248	291	337
285	130	157	188	223	263	307	355
310	140	168	200	237	278	324	373
335	149	179	213	251	294	341	391

ECG SHOWS ENLARGED HEART (LVH)

SBP	105	120	135	150	165	180	195
Chol.							
185	118	142	170	203	240	282	328
210	126	152	182	216	255	298	345
235	135	162	194	230	270	315	363
260	144	173	206	244	286	332	381
285	154	184	219	258	302	349	400
310	164	196	233	273	318	367	419
335	175	209	247	289	336	385	438

SBP	105	120	135	150	165	180	195
Chol.							
185	209	246	289	335	385	437	491
210	222	261	305	353	404	457	511
235	235	277	322	371	423	476	530
260	250	292	339	389	442	495	549
285	265	309	357	408	461	515	569
310	280	326	375	427	480	534	588
335	296	343	393	446	500	554	606

have glucose intolerance. At these average values the probability of developing cardiovascular disease in eight years is 119/1000.

TABLE 2O. PROBABILITY (PER 1,000) OF DEVELOPING CARDIOVASCULAR

DOES NOT SMOKE CIGARETTES

NO ENLARGED HEART BY ECG

	SBP	105	120	135	150	165	180	195
	Chol.							
GLUCOSE	185		70	85	104	126	152	182	216
INTOLERANCE	210		73	89	109	132	158	189	225
ABSENT	235		77	94	114	137	165	197	234
	260		81	98	119	144	172	205	243
	285		84	103	124	150	180	214	252
	310		88	108	130	157	187	223	262
	335		93	113	136	163	195	232	272

	SBP	105	120	135	150	165	180	195
	Chol.							
GLUCOSE	185	129	156	187	222	261	305	353
INTOLERANCE	210	135	163	194	231	271	316	364
PRESENT	235	141	170	202	240	281	327	376
	260	148	177	211	249	292	338	388
	285	154	185	219	259	302	350	401
	310	161	192	228	269	313	362	413
	335	168	200	237	279	324	373	425

ECG SHOWS ENLARGED HEART (LVH)

	SBP	105	120	135	150	165	180	195
	Chol.							
GLUCOSE	185	153	183	217	257	300	347	398
INTOLERANCE	210	159	191	226	266	311	359	410
ABSENT	235	166	199	235	276	322	371	422
	260	174	207	245	287	333	383	435
	285	181	215	254	297	344	395	447
	310	189	224	264	308	356	407	460
	335	197	233	273	319	368	419	473

	SBP	105	120	135	150	165	180	195
	Chol.							
GLUCOSE	185	263	307	355	406	459	513	566
INTOLERANCE	210	273	318	367	418	471	525	579
PRESENT	235	283	329	378	430	484	538	591
	260	294	340	390	443	497	551	604
	285	304	352	403	456	510	563	616
	310	315	364	415	468	522	576	628
	335	326	375	427	481	535	588	640

*Framingham women aged 65 years have an average SBP of 151 mm. Hg and an average serum cholesterol of 269 mg.%; 23% smoke cigarettes, 3.1% have definite LVH by ECG, and 9.0%

SMOKES CIGARETTES

NO ENLARGED HEART BY ECG

SBP	105	120	135	150	165	180	195
Chol.							
185	73	89	108	130	157	188	223
210	76	93	113	136	164	195	232
235	80	97	118	142	171	204	241
260	84	102	123	149	178	212	250
285	88	106	129	155	186	221	260
310	92	111	135	162	193	229	270
335	96	117	141	169	202	239	280

SBP	105	120	135	150	165	180	195
Chol.							
185	134	161	193	229	269	313	362
210	140	168	201	238	279	325	374
235	146	175	209	247	289	336	386
260	153	183	218	257	300	347	398
285	159	191	226	266	311	359	410
310	166	199	235	276	322	371	422
335	174	207	245	287	333	383	435

ECG SHOWS ENLARGED HEART (LVH)

SBP	105	120	135	150	165	180	195
Chol.							
185	158	189	224	264	308	356	407
210	165	197	233	274	319	368	420
235	172	205	243	284	330	380	432
260	179	213	252	295	342	392	445
285	187	222	262	306	353	404	457
310	195	231	272	317	365	417	470
335	203	240	282	328	377	429	483

SBP	105	120	135	150	165	180	195
Chol.							
185	271	315	364	415	469	523	576
210	281	326	376	428	481	535	589
235	291	338	388	440	494	548	601
260	302	349	400	453	507	561	613
285	313	361	412	465	519	573	625
310	324	373	425	478	532	585	637
335	335	385	437	491	545	598	649

have glucose intolerance. At these average values the probability of developing cardiovascular disease in eight years is 160/1000.

TABLE 2P. PROBABILITY (PER 1,000) OF DEVELOPING CARDIOVASCULAR

DOES NOT SMOKE CIGARETTES

NO ENLARGED HEART BY ECG

	SBP	105	120	135	150	165	180	195
	Chol.							
GLUCOSE	185	90	110	133	160	191	227	267
INTOLERANCE	210	92	112	136	163	195	231	272
ABSENT	235	94	115	139	166	199	235	276
	260	97	117	141	170	202	240	281
	285	99	120	144	173	206	244	286
	310	101	122	147	177	210	249	291
	335	103	125	150	180	214	253	296

	SBP	105	120	135	150	165	180	195
	Chol.							
GLUCOSE	185	164	196	233	273	318	367	419
INTOLERANCE	210	168	200	237	278	324	373	425
PRESENT	235	171	204	241	283	329	378	430
	260	174	208	246	288	334	384	436
	285	178	212	250	293	340	390	442
	310	181	216	255	298	345	395	448
	335	185	220	259	303	351	401	454

ECG SHOWS ENLARGED HEART (LVH)

	SBP	105	120	135	150	165	180	195
	Chol.							
GLUCOSE	185	192	228	269	313	362	413	466
INTOLERANCE	210	196	233	273	318	367	419	472
ABSENT	235	200	237	278	324	373	425	478
	260	204	241	283	329	378	430	484
	285	208	246	288	334	384	436	490
	310	212	250	293	340	390	442	496
	335	216	255	298	345	395	448	502

	SBP	105	120	135	150	165	180	195
	Chol.							
GLUCOSE	185	320	369	421	474	528	582	633
INTOLERANCE	210	326	375	427	480	534	588	639
PRESENT	235	331	380	433	486	540	593	644
	260	336	386	439	492	546	599	650
	285	342	392	444	498	552	605	655
	310	347	398	450	504	558	611	661
	335	353	403	456	510	564	616	666

*Framingham women aged 70 years have an average SBP of 158 mm. Hg and an average serum cholesterol of 267 mg.%; 15% smoke cigarettes, 1.4% have definite LVH by ECG, and 8.1%

SMOKES CIGARETTES

NO ENLARGED HEART BY ECG

Chol. \ SBP	105	120	135	150	165	180	195
185	94	114	138	165	197	234	275
210	96	116	140	169	201	238	280
235	98	119	143	172	205	243	284
260	100	121	146	175	209	247	289
285	102	124	149	179	213	251	294
310	104	126	152	182	217	256	299
335	107	129	155	186	221	261	304

Chol. \ SBP	105	120	135	150	165	180	195
185	170	203	240	281	327	376	428
210	173	206	244	286	332	382	434
235	177	210	249	291	338	388	440
260	180	214	253	296	343	393	446
285	184	219	258	301	349	399	452
310	187	223	262	306	354	405	458
335	191	227	267	311	360	411	464

ECG SHOWS ENLARGED HEART (LVH)

Chol. \ SBP	105	120	135	150	165	180	195
185	199	235	277	322	371	423	476
210	203	240	281	327	376	428	482
235	206	244	286	332	382	434	488
260	210	249	291	338	388	440	494
285	214	253	296	343	393	446	500
310	219	258	301	349	399	452	506
335	223	262	306	354	405	458	512

Chol. \ SBP	105	120	135	150	165	180	195
185	329	378	431	484	538	591	642
210	334	384	436	490	544	597	648
235	340	390	442	496	550	603	653
260	345	396	448	502	556	609	659
285	351	401	454	508	562	614	664
310	356	407	460	514	568	620	670
335	362	413	466	520	574	626	675

have glucose intolerance. At these average values the probability of developing cardiovascular disease in eight years is 199/1000.

Glossary

Angina pectoris. Chest pains that result from decreased blood flow because of narrowing of the coronary arteries caused by atherosclerosis.

Angiography. A technique that permits visualization of blood vessels by using X-ray motion pictures after injection of a radiopaque dye. This general term includes arteries and veins, unlike *arteriography,* which is limited to arteries.

Aorta. The main artery of the body; it gives off all the arterial branches that nourish the heart and major organs.

Arteriography. The process of visualizing the boundary of an artery by taking X-ray motion pictures after a radiopaque dye is injected.

Arterioles. Small arteries that have a muscular wall. The arterioles branch into smaller blood vessels known as capillaries.

Arteriosclerosis. A disease of the arteries that is often known as hardening of the arteries. It is often used interchangeably with atherosclerosis.

Artery. A muscular blood vessel that carries blood away from the heart to the tissues. It is composed of an outer lining called the adventitia, a muscular middle layer consisting of smooth muscle fibers, and an inner lining called the intima.

Asymptomatic. A term describing a patient who has no symptoms.

Atheroma. A deposit of fat cholesterol and smooth muscle cells within the inner layer (intima) of an artery.

Atherosclerosis. A disease that is characterized by the deposition of fat and cholesterol within the inner wall of an artery.

Atherosclerotic coronary-artery disease. A type of narrowing of the arteries caused by the deposition of lipid within the inner wall of the coronary arteries.

Atrium. The thin-walled heart chambers that receive the blood returning from the body (right atrium) and the lungs (left atrium).

Beta blockers. Drugs inhibiting stimulatory impulses to the heart. Beta blocks result in a slower, less forceful heart contraction.

Beta stimulation of the heart. Beta stimulation results in an increased heart rate and increased force of cardiac contraction.

242

Bifurcation. The junction at which an artery branches into two subdivisions.

Brand name. The name of a drug that is chosen and advertised by a specific manufacturer. Compare *generic name.*

Calorie. Unit of energy. When used to describe food energy, it is a measure of the body's energy needs. A calorie is the amount of energy necessary to raise the temperature of 1 gram of water 1° C, under 1 atmosphere of pressure.

Capillaries. The smallest blood vessels, which connect arteries and veins. Capillaries have very thin walls that allow oxygen and nutrients to pass easily into surrounding cells.

Cardiac. Pertaining to the heart.

Cardiovascular. Pertaining to the heart and blood vessels.

Cholesterol. A fatty material found only in animal tissues and absent from fruits, vegetables, and cereals. It can be manufactured by the body.

Circulatory. Refers to the flow of blood through the heart, veins, arteries, and capillaries.

Circumflex coronary artery. One of two major branches of the left coronary artery.

Collagen. A fibrous protein constituent of connective tissue.

Collateral circulation. Developed connections for circulation around an arterial obstruction.

Congestive heart failure. The inability of the heart to pump enough blood. It results in congestion of the liver, lungs, and other organs with blood that has been dammed.

Coronary arteriography. The study of the anatomy of the coronary arteries by using a radiopaque dye injected by a special tube (catheter).

Coronary artery. An artery that arises from the aorta and nourishes the heart. The arteries encircle the heart (*coronary* is derived from the Latin *corono,* meaning "to encircle").

Diastole. The phase of the heart's cycle that occurs during the relaxation of the heart muscle.

Digoxin. A form of digitalis, a drug that strengthens the contractions of the heart.

Diuretic. A drug that increases the amount of urine flow.

Edema. The presence of abnormally large amounts of fluid in the tissues outside the blood vessels. Commonly it is first noted in the legs, though it can occur in the lungs.

Electrocardiogram. A recording of the electrical activity of the heart.

Etiology. The cause of a disease.

Generic name. The scientific (as opposed to commercial) name of a drug. Compare *brand name.*

Genetic. Relating to the hereditary material received from parents.

Hypercholesterolemia. Abnormal elevation of cholesterol in the blood. It can be genetically determined or the result of dietary intake.

Hyperlipoproteinemia. A condition of excessive levels of blood fats, cholesterol, or triglyceride in the blood.

Hypertension. An elevation of the blood pressure within the arteries.

Hypertriglyceridemia. Excessive levels of triglyceride in the blood.

Hypertrophy. Enlargement of an organ.

Hypoxia. Inadequate oxygen levels in the arterial blood.

Incidence. The frequency with which a specific disease occurs within a population.

Intermittent claudication. Symptoms of pain in the legs caused by a lack of oxygen due to atherosclerotic narrowing of the arteries that nourish the legs. The pain is induced by walking and relieved by rest.

Intima. The innermost layer of the arterial wall.

Ischemia. Inadequate oxygen to the tissues.

Left anterior descending artery. One of the two main branches of the left main coronary artery.

Lesion. A structural abnormality.

Lipids. Fatty organic compounds that include both cholesterol and triglyceride. Lipids are found in the blood and tissues.

Lipoproteins. A combination of protein and lipid that is soluble in the blood.

Lumen. The passageway within a blood vessel.

Maximum heart rate. The highest heart rate that can be achieved with maximal effort. It is usually estimated as 220 minus the subject's age (i.e., at age 40 the maximum heart rate would be 220 minus 40, or 180 beats per minute).

Media. The middle layer of an artery; it contains smooth muscle cells.

Mitral valve. The valve separating the left atrium from the left ventricle.

Myocardial infarction. A heart attack, manifested by death of a portion of the heart muscle.

Myocardium. The muscular wall of the heart.

Nitroglycerin. A drug that relieves the pain of angina pectoris promptly. It is usually taken by permitting a tablet to dissolve underneath the tongue. It can also be used as an ointment.

Noninvasive. Relating to any procedure that does not involve injection or insertion of foreign chemicals or tubes into the body.

Pericardium. The lining that surrounds the heart.

Plaque. An area of localized atherosclerosis that occurs on the inner surface of an artery and extends into the lumen. Plaques have a yellow color because they contain lipids.

Plasma. The fluid portion of the blood. It remains after the cellular elements have been removed by centrifugation.

Platelet. A disclike particle that participates in the clotting of blood.

Pneumatic cuff (sphygmomanometer). A rubber bladder that is inflated with air in order to constrict the artery in the arm. It is used to measure the blood pressure.

Polyunsaturated fats. Fats of vegetable origin that contain space for additional hydrogen atoms on their molecules. They do not harden at room temperature.

Propranolol. A beta-blocking agent used to treat angina, high blood pressure, and abnormal heart rhythms.

Pulmonary edema. The accumulation of excessive fluid in the lungs, usually because of heart failure.

Radiopaque dye. A material that absorbs X rays so that they can be used to outline a structure.

Retina. The inner lining of the eyeball.

Rheumatic fever. An inflammatory disease that follows infection with certain streptococcal bacteria and may damage heart valves and heart muscle.

Saphenous veins. The large veins of the legs.

Saphenous vein bypass surgery. An operation for coronary-artery narrowing. It consists of removing a vein from the saphenous vein in the leg and attaching it to the aorta above the obstruction of the coronary artery and to the disease-free segment of the coronary artery below the obstruction.

Saturated fats. Fats, usually of animal origin, that contain all the hydrogen they can accept. They harden at room temperature.

Systole. The phase of the heart's cycle that occurs during the contraction of the heart muscle.

Target heart rate. The heart rate that should be achieved during exercise in order to provide a training effect. Physical fitness requires a minimum of 70–80 percent of the maximal heart rate during exercise.

Thrombus. A clot occluding a blood vessel, produced by coagulation of the blood.

Triglyceride. A fat containing glycerin and three fatty acids. It can be of animal or vegetable origin and can be eaten preformed or be manufactured in the body.

Type-A personality. A hard-driving, time-conscious person.

Type-B personality. A person who is lacking in time consciousness, speaks slowly, and does not attempt to do two things at the same time.

Ultrasound. A diagnostic technique that uses sound waves that are bounced off the heart's surfaces to outline structures.

Uric acid. A by-product of certain protein substances found in the blood and urine. Elevated levels are found in gout, a painful type of arthritis.

Vascular. Relating to the blood vessels.

Vein. A thin-walled blood vessel that carries blood back to the heart.

Ventricle. The two large pumping chambers of the heart.

Ventricular fibrillation. An irregular heart rhythm in which blood is not pumped and the circulation fails abruptly.

Bibliography

Anderson, J. T.; Grand, F.; and Keys, A. "Cholesterol-Lowering Diets." *Journal of American Dietetic Association* 62 (1973): 133.

Angelico, R. "Outlines of Dietary Prevention of Atherosclerosis." *Advances in Experimental Medicine and Biology* 60 (1975): 171.

Anguelles, A. E.; Martinez, M. A.; Hoffman, C.; Ortiz, G. A.; and Chekherdemian, M. "Corticoadrenal and Adrenergic Overactivity and Hyperlipidemia in Prolonged Emotional Stress." *Hormones* 3 (1972): 167.

Armstrong, M. L.; Warren, E. D.; and Connor, W. E. "Regression of Coronary Athermatosis in Rhesus Monkeys." *Circulation Research* 27 (1970): 59.

Aronow, W. S.; Allen, W. H.; and Cristofaro, D. D. "Response of Patients and Physicians to Mass Screening for Coronary Risk Factors." *Circulation* 52 (1975): 586.

————; and Ungermann, S. "Follow-up of Mass Screening for Coronary Risk Factors in 1817 Adults." *Circulation* 51 (1975): 1038.

————; Ungermann, S.; Wan, M. K.; Chun, G. M.; Leik, S. W.; and Savitz, S. P. "Mass Screening for Coronary Risk Factors in 2524 Asymptomatic Adults." *Journal of American Geriatrics Society* 23 (1975): 121.

Banks, D. C.; Raftery, E. B.; and Oran, S. "Clinical Significance of Coronary Arteriogram." *British Heart Journal* 33 (1971): 863.

Barndt, R., and Blankenhorn, D. H. "Regression of Femoral Atherosclerosis in Man." *Internal Medical News* 9 (1976): 1.

————; Crawford, D. W.; and Brooks, S. H. "Regression and Progression of Early Femoral Atherosclerosis in Treated Hyperlipidemic Patients." *Annals of Internal Medicine* 86 (1976): 139.

————; Crawford, D. W.; Zenphenyi, T.; Kanabus, W.; Richardson, R. P.; and Brooks, S. H. "In vivo Evidence of Atherosclerotic Regression with Risk Factor Reduction in Hyperlipidemic Patients." *American College of Physicians Annual Session* (1976): 45.

Basta, L. L.; Williams, C.; Kioschos, J. M.; and Spector, A. A. "Regression of Athero-sclerosis Stenosing Lesions of the Renal Arteries and Spontaneous Cure of Systemic Hypertension through Control of Hyperlipidemia." *American Journal of Medicine* 61 (1976): 420.

Ben-Zui, J.; Hildner, F. J.; Javier, R. P.; Fester, A.; and Samet, P. "Progression of Coronary Artery Disease." *American Journal of Cardiology* 34 (1974): 295.

Bierenbaum, M. L. "The Five-Year Experience with Modified Fat Diets on Younger Men with Coronary Heart Disease." *Circulation* 42 (1970): 943.

———; Fleischman, A. O.; Raichelson, R. O.; Hayton, T.; and Watson, P. B. "Ten-Year Experience of Modified Fat Diets on Younger Men with Coronary Heart Disease." *Lancet* 23 (1973): 1404.

Blackburn, H. "Contrasting Professional Views on Atherosclerosis and Coronary Disease." *New England Journal of Medicine* 292 (1975): 105.

Buchwald, H.; Moore, R. B.; and Varco, R. L. "Surgical Treatment of Hyperlipidemia." *Circulation* 46, Supp. 1 (1974): 33.

———; Varco, R. L.; Moore, R. B.; and Schwartz, M. Z. "Surgical Treatment of Hyperlipidemia." *Current Problems in Surgery* 20 (1975): 1.

Christakis, G.; Rinsler, S. H.; Archer, M.; Winslow, G.; Jempel, S.; Stephenson, H.; Friedman, G.; Fein, H.; and Kraus, A. "Prevention of Coronary Heart Disease —A Seven-Year Report." *American Journal of Public Health* 56 (1966): 299.

Cohn, K.; Sukai, J. F.; and Langston, M. F. "Effect of Clofibrate on Progression of Coronary Disease." *American Heart Journal* 89 (1975): 591.

Connor, W. E., and Connor, S. "The Key Role of Nutritional Factors in the Prevention of Coronary Heart Disease." *Preventive Medicine* 1 (1972): 49.

Dayton, S.; Pearce, M. L.; Hashimoto, S.; Dixon, W. J.; and Tomeyasu, V. "A Controlled Clinical Trial of a Diet High in Unsaturated Fat in Preventing Complications of Atherosclerosis." *Circulation* 39, Supp. 2 (1969): 1.

Deutscher, S. "Some Factors Influencing the Distribution of Premature Death from Coronary Heart Disease in Nova Scotia." *American Journal of Public Health* 63 (1973): 150.

Eggen, D. A.; Strong, J. P.; and Newman, W. P., III. "Regression of Diet—Induced Fatty Streaks in Rhesus Monkeys." *Laboratory Investigation* 31 (1974): 292.

Gensini, G. G., and Kelly, A. E. "Incidence and Progression of Coronary Artery Disease." *Archives of Internal Medicine* 129 (1972): 814.

Gresham, G. A. "Is Atherome a Reversible Lesion?" *Atherosclerosis* 23 (1976): 379.

Haskell, W. L.; Stern, M. P.; Wood, P. D.; Brown, W. B.; Garquheir, J. W.; and Maccoby, N. "A Multifactor Education Campaign to Reduce Cardiovascular Risk in Three Communities." *Circulation* 50, Supp. 3 (1974): 101.

Keyes, A., ed. "Coronary Heart Disease in Seven Countries." *Circulation* 41, Supp. 1 (1970): 1.

Kimbiris, D.; Lavine, P.; Van den Browk, H.; Najmi, M.; and Likoff, W. "Devolution-ary Pattern of Coronary Atherosclerosis in Patients with Angina Pectoris." *American Journal of Cardiology* 33 (1974): 7.

Know, E. G. "New Etiologies for Ischemic Heart Disease." *American Heart Journal* 88 (1974): 809.

Lofland, H. B.; St. Clair, R. W.; and Clarkson, T. B. "Biochemical Changes in the Artery Wall During Genesis and Regression of Atheromatous Lesions." *Advances in Experimental Medicine and Biology* 26 (1972): 91.

Meyer, A. J., and Henderson, J. B. "Multiple Risk Factor Reduction in the Prevention of Cardiovascular Disease." *Preventive Medicine* 5 (1974): 237.

Miettinen, M.; Turpeinen, O.; Darvonen, M. J.; Elosuo, R.; and Paavilainen, E. "Effect of Cholesterol-Lowering Diet on Mortality from Coronary Heart Disease and Other Causes: A Twelve-Year Clinical Trial in Men and Women." *Lancet* 21 (1972): 835.

Morris, D. C.; Jurst, J. W.; and Lougue, R. B. "Myocardial Infarction in Young Women." *American Journal of Cardiology* 38 (1976): 299.

Nash, D. T. "The Erysichthon Syndrome, Accelerated Vascular Disease Due to Dietary Hyperlipidemia." Paper presented at American College of Cardiology annual meeting, Las Vegas, March 9, 1977.

———; Caldwell, N.; and Ancona, D. "Accelerated Coronary Artery Disease Arterio-graphically Proven." *New York State Journal of Medicine* 74 (1974): 947.

———; Gensini, G.; Simon, H.; Arno, T.; Nash, S. D. "Erysichthon Syndrome, Progression of Coronary Atherosclerosis and Dietary Hyperlipidemia." *Circulation* 56 (1977): 363.

Nitter-Hauge, S., and Enge, I. "Relation Between Blood Lipid Levels and Angiograph-ically Evaluated Obstructions in Coronary Arteries." *British Heart Journal* 35 (1973): 791.

Oliver, M. "Dietary Cholesterol, Plasma Cholesterol and Coronary Heart Disease." *British Heart Journal* 38 (1976): 214.

Page, I. H.; Berrettoni, A. B.; and Sones, F. M. "Prediction of Coronary Heart Disease Based on Clinical Suspicion, Age, Total Cholesterol, and Triglyceride." *Circulation* 42 (1970): 635.

Pritchard, R. W. "Recent Advances in Molecular Pathology, Regression of Athero-sclerosis—A Perspective." *Experimental Molecular Pathology* 20 (1974): 407.

Punsar, S.; Erametsa, O.; Karvonen, M. J.; Ryhanen, A.; Hilska, P.; and Vornamo, H. "Coronary Heart Disease and Drinking Water: A Search in Two Finnish Male Cohorts for Epidemiologic Evidence of a Water Factor." *Journal of Chronic Diseases* 28 (1975): 259.

Rinsler, S. H. "Primary Prevention of Coronary Heart Disease by Diet." *Academy of Medicine* 44 (1968): 936.

Ross, R., and Glomset, J. A. "The Pathogenesis of Atherosclerosis." *Journal of English Medicine* 295 (1976): 369.

Ross, R., and Harker, L. "Hyperlipidemia and Atherosclerosis." *Science* 193 (1976): 1094.

Schroeder, H. A. "The Role of Trace Elements in Cardiovascular Diseases." *Medical Clinics of North America* 58 (1974): 381.

Silverstone, T. *Obesity: Its Pathogenesis and Management.* Acton, Mass.: Publishing Science Group, 1975.

Small, D. M., and Shipley, G. G. "Physical-Chemical Basis of Lipid Deposition in Atherosclerosis." *Science* 185 (1974): 222.

Somogyi, J. C. "Prevention of Atherosclerosis by Diet: Present State and Conclusions." *Advances in Experimental Medicine and Biology* 60 (1975): 205.

Stamler, J. "Primary Prevention of Sudden Coronary Death." *Circulation* 51, Supp. 3 (1975): 258.

Stanton, G. A. "Annotations: The Cause of Arterial Disease." *American Heart Journal* 87 (1974): 796.

Steinburg, D. "Planning the Type II Coronary Primary Prevention Trial of the Lipid Research Clinics (U.S.A.)." *Advances in Experimental Medicine and Biology* 63 (1975): 417.

Stunkard, A., and McLaren-Hume, M. "The Results of Treatment for Obesity." *Archives of Internal Medicine* 103 (1959): 79.

Turner, R., and Ball, K. "The Cardiologist's Responsibility for Preventing Coronary Heart Disease." *American Heart Journal* 91 (1976): 139.

Turpeinen, O.; Miettiren, M.; Karuonen, M. II.; Roire, P.; Pekkarinen, M.; Lehtosuo, E. J.; and Alivirta, P. "Blood Lipids and Primary Coronary Events: The Effect of Diet Modification." *Minnesota Medicine* 52 (1969): 1947.

————. "Dietary Prevention of Coronary Heart Disease: Long-term Experiment, Observations on Male Subjects." *American Journal of Clinical Nutrition* 21 (1968): 255.

Vedin, J. A.; Wilhelmsson, C.; Elmfeldt, D.; Tibblin, G.; Wilhelmsen, L.; and Werko, L. "Sudden Death: Identification of High-Risk Groups." *American Heart Journal* 86 (1973): 124.

Welch, C. C.; Proudfet, W. L.; Sones, F. M.; Shirley, E. K.; Sheldon, W. C.; and Razavi, M. "Cinecoronary Arteriography in Young Men." *Circulation* 42 (1970): 647.

West, R. R.; Lloyd, S.; and Roberts, C. J. "Mortality from Ischaemic Heart Disease—Association with Weather." *Brit. J. Prev. Soc. Med.* 27 (1973): 36.

Wilhelmsen, L.; Sanne, H.; Elmfeldt, D.; Grimby, G.; Tibblin, G.; and Wedel, H. "A Controlled Trial of Physical Training after Myocardial Infarction: Effects on Risk Factors, Nonfatal Reinfarction and Death." *Preventive Medicine* 4 (1975): 491.

Wilson, N. *Obesity.* Philadelphia: F. A. Davis, 1969.

Wissler, R. W., and Vesselenovitch, D. "The Effects of Feeding Various Dietary Fats on the Development and Regression of Hypercholesterolemia and Atherosclerosis." *Advanced Experimental Medical Biology* 60 (1975): 65.

Woffram, G. "Reversibility of Lipid Deposition." *Nutrition and Metabolism* 15 (1973): 141.

Wright, I. S. "Correct Levels of Serum Cholesterol." *Journal of the American Medical Association* 236 (1976): 261.

Zilversmit, D. B. "Mechanism of Cholesterol Accumulation in the Arterial Wall." *American Journal of Cardiology* 35 (1975): 559.

Index